HOW TO SURVIVE
IN ANAESTHESIA

HOW TO SURVIVE IN ANAESTHESIA

P NEVILLE ROBINSON MB ChB FRCA
Department of Anaesthesia
Northwick Park and St Mark's Hospitals
Harrow, Middlesex

and

GEORGE M HALL MB BS PhD FRCA
Department of Anaesthesia
St George's Hospital Medical School
London

BMJ
Publishing
Group

First published 1997
Reprinted 1999
by the BMJ Publishing Group, BMA House, Tavistock Square,
London WC1H 9JR

British Library Cataloguing in Publication Data

A catalogue record for this book is available from the
British Library

ISBN 0-7279-1066-3

Typeset, printed and bound in Great Britain by
Latimer Trend & Company Ltd, Plymouth

Contents

Part III Passing the gas

List of boxes

Preface

If you are a trained anaesthetist, you should not be reading this. If you have just started anaesthesia, congratulations on your choice; you have joined the most interesting specialty in medicine which contains some of the most intelligent, well-adjusted consultants to be found in hospitals (we can think of at least two). In your first few weeks of anaesthesia you will be given much advice, some of which may even be good, and will be influenced by the current issues affecting the specialty. It is easy to believe that audit, high dependency units, acute pain teams, *et cetera*, are areas of essential knowledge for the newcomer. They are not. They only become relevant when you are capable of conducting a safe anaesthetic. We hope that this short book will help trainees in the first year of anaesthesia by emphasising basic principles and key concepts. Full explanations have been left for "proper" textbooks.

We thank the many trainees who over the years have kept us entertained, enthused, sometimes informed, occasionally frightened, and whose ingenuity in devising new mistakes never ceased to amaze.

P Neville Robinson
George M Hall

Part I
Nuts and bolts

The first section of this book deals with two fundamental aspects of anaesthetic practice: the airway and vascular access. General anaesthesia has been summarised by the simple phrase *put up a drip, put down a tube and give plenty of oxygen.* Many anaesthetists resent this glib description of their work, but it does have the virtue of emphasising the importance of venous cannulation and control of the airway, which are essential for the safe conduct of anaesthesia. Difficulties arise in anaesthesia when one of these fundamental areas is not secure and, if both fail, then disaster is close at hand.

Therefore, in the first 10 chapters we concentrate on evaluation and control of the airway, the anaesthetic machine and circuits, basic anaesthetic monitoring, vascular access, and the choice of intravenous fluids. We have not given detailed instructions on how to undertake the practical procedures. There is no substitute for careful instruction from a senior anaesthetist as part of the anaesthetic procedure. At the start of training the application of physiology and pharmacology to anaesthesia is exciting, and knowledge of the equipment may seem mundane and even boring. It is imperative that you have a basic understanding of the equipment you use—failure to do so will put the patient at risk.

1: Evaluation of the airway

Control of the airway is fundamental for safe anaesthetic practice and careful assessment must be undertaken preoperatively. This is carried out logically as summarised in Box 1.1.

Box 1.1 Assessment of the airway

- History

- Symptoms

- Examination
  - anatomy and variants
  - medical conditions
  - specific assessment
    - Mallampati scoring system
    - Wilson risk factor scoring system
    - thyromental distance

- Other tests

History

Any previous anaesthetic history must be obtained. Information about difficulties with endotracheal intubation may be found in old anaesthetic records. Previous successful intubation is not an indicator of its ease. Some patients wear Medic-alert bracelets stating their anaesthetic difficulties, whilst others with major problems know nothing about such problems.

Symptoms

Upper airway obstruction may be found in patients with stridor, dysphagia, and hoarseness.

Examination and clinical tests

Normal anatomy and its variants

Some patients appear anatomically normal and yet are difficult, or impossible, to intubate. These patients cause anaesthetists unexpected problems and we have had the occasional experience of casually starting an apparently normal laryngoscopy, only to have the sinking feeling associated with complete failure to visualise the larynx. It is much better to anticipate a difficulty than encounter one unexpectedly. Some anatomical factors that make airway control and intubation difficult are listed in Box 1.2.

Box 1.2   Anatomical features of difficult airway control and intubation

- Short immobile neck
- Full set of teeth, buck teeth
- High arch palate
- Poor mouth opening
- Receding mandible
- Inability to sublux the jaw (forward protrusion of the lower incisors beyond the upper incisors)

Medical conditions

Medical problems associated with increased difficulty of endotracheal intubation are listed in Box 1.3.

Box 1.3   Medical features of difficult airway intubation

- Congenital: rare

- Acquired
  - traumatic: fractures of mandible and cervical spine
  - infection: epiglottitis, dental or facial abscess
  - endocrine: thyroid enlargement, acromegaly, obesity
  - neoplasia: tongue, neck, mouth, radiotherapy
  - inflammatory: ankylosing spondylitis, rheumatoid arthritis
  - pregnancy

Specific assessment

Three clinical tests to assess the airway are in common use.

Modified Mallampati scoring system

This predicts about 50% of difficult intubations. The test can be performed with the patient in the upright or supine position. It is based upon the visibility of the pharyngeal structures with the mouth open as wide as possible (Figure 1.1). Patients are classified as follows:

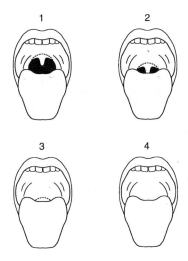

FIG 1.1—*Structures seen on opening of mouth for Mallampati Grades 1–4*

- Grade 1: faucial pillars, soft palate and uvula visible
- Grade 2: (faucial pillars) soft palate visible, but uvula masked by the base of the tongue
- Grade 3: soft palate only visible
- Grade 4: soft palate not visible.

Patients in Grades 3 and 4 are considered difficult to intubate and those in Grades 1 and 2 are considered feasible intubations. It is important to realise that this system is *not* infallible and patients in Grade 2 are sometimes not able to be intubated.

Wilson risk factor scoring system (Box 1.4)

Five anatomical features are assessed and a total risk score of >2 is said to predict 75% of difficult intubations.

Box 1.4 Wilson risk factor scoring system for difficult intubation

Risk factor	Score	Criteria
Weight	0	<90 kg
	1	90–110 kg
	2	>110 kg
Head and neck movement	0	>90°
	1	about 90°
	2	<90°
Jaw movement	0	incisor gap >5 cm or subluxation >0
	1	incisor gap <5 cm and subluxation =0
	2	incisor gap <5 cm and subluxation <0
Receding mandible	0	normal
	1	moderate
	2	severe
Buck teeth	0	normal
	1	moderate
	2	severe

Thyromental distance

The thyromental distance is the distance from the thyroid cartilage to the mental prominence when the neck is extended fully (Figure 1.2). In the absence of other anatomical factors, if the distance is >6·5 cm, problems should not occur with intubation. A distance of <6 cm suggests laryngoscopy

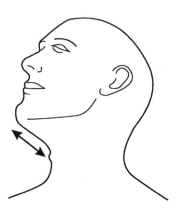

FIG 1.2—*Line shows the thyromental distance from the thyroid cartilage to the tip of the chin*

will be impossible and for distances between 6–6·5 cm, laryngoscopy is considered difficult, but possible. This measurement may predict up to 75% of difficult intubations.

Other tests

Indirect laryngoscopy and various X-ray procedures are occasionally used. With X-rays the effective mandibular length has been compared with the posterior depth of the mandible; a ratio of >3·6 may be associated with a difficult intubation. A decreased distance between the occiput and the spinous process of C1 is also reported as associated with difficulties with laryngoscopy. We have found these tests to be of limited value.

Conclusion

The airway must be assessed before any anaesthetic procedure is embarked upon. Airway control and endotracheal intubation is occasionally difficult, or even impossible, in anatomically normal people. An assessment from the patient's history, symptoms and medical conditions, combined with careful clinical examination, will help avoid most, but not all, unexpectedly difficult intubations.

2: Control of the airway

The novice anaesthetist must learn rapidly the skills of airway control.

Position

The patient must be correctly positioned. This is achieved by elevating the head by about the height of a pillow to flex the neck. The head is extended on the cervical spine and the mandible lifted forward to stop obstruction from the tongue and other pharyngeal structures that lose their tone under anaesthesia. This position is commonly referred to as "sniffing the early morning air", a practice not to be recommended in a modern urban environment.

Methods

There are four methods of airway control which are used for the purpose of ensuring unobstructed gas exchange (Box 2.1).

Box 2.1   Methods of airway control

- Facemask and Guedel airway
- Laryngeal mask
- Endotracheal tube
- Tracheostomy

Face mask

The mask is designed to fit snugly over the patient's nose and mouth. However, gas often leaks round the side of the mask in edentulous patients. An obstructed airway may be relieved by the insertion of an oropharyngeal airway (Guedel airway) or by a nasopharyngeal airway. Guedel airways are sized from 0 to 4, with a size 3 used for adult females and 4 for adult males. Nasopharyngeal airways can cause haemorrhage, unless they are inserted very gently, which may further threaten the airway.

Laryngeal mask

This was developed from the concept that the anaesthetic face mask could, instead of being applied to the face, be altered and positioned over the laryngeal opening (Figure 2.1). It is inserted using a blind technique and provides a patent airway for spontaneous breathing; it is used occasionally for ventilation and management of difficult intubation. The experienced anaesthetist can pass a 6·0 mm cuffed endotracheal tube, gum elastic bougie or fibreoptic laryngoscope through the laryngeal mask. A black line is present on the tube which ensures correct orientation of the mask. The sizes are 2 and $2\frac{1}{2}$ for children, 3 for adult females and 4 for adult males.

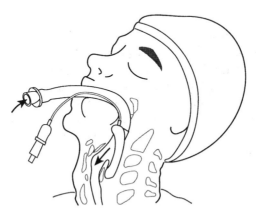

FIG 2.1—*Laryngeal mask correctly positioned before inflation, with the tip of the mask in the base of the hypopharynx*

The main advantage of this technique is that the anaesthetist has both hands free to undertake other tasks. The laryngeal mask permits the measurement of the oxygen, carbon dioxide and volatile anaesthetic concentration in the expired gas.

The mask does *not* prevent gastric aspiration occurring, is not suitable for emergency anaesthesia, and incorrect positioning can occur which may lead to airway obstruction. This is often due to folding back of the epiglottis as it is pushed down by the mask during insertion and occurs in about 10% of patients.

Endotracheal tubes

A cuffed endotracheal tube, once inserted into the trachea, maintains airway patency and minimises gastric aspiration into the lungs. All endotracheal tubes have information written upon the tube (Figure 2.2). A novice anaesthetist is expected to be able to provide a detailed description of the information on an endotracheal tube: it is a basic tool of the trade! The tube is inserted by the laryngoscope being held in the left hand and the blade passed into the right side of the mouth. The tongue is then pushed to the left as the blade is passed down the tongue and inserted

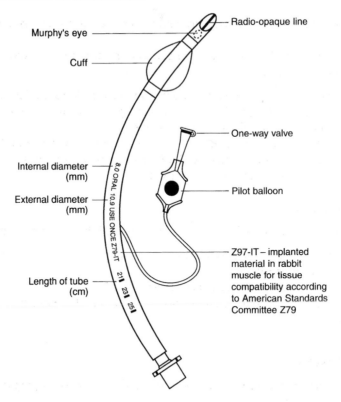

FIG 2.2—*Typical endotracheal tube*

anterior to the epiglottis in the vallecula. Elevation of the whole laryngoscope will facilitate a clear view of the glottic opening (Figure 2.3).

Tips to aid insertion of the endotracheal tube include:

- the use of a gum elastic bougie inserted through the larynx with the tube passed over it;

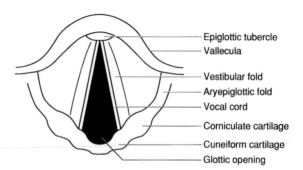

FIG 2.3—*View of the larynx obtained before intubation*

- the application of pressure externally over the larynx to bring it into view;
- a "helping finger" from an assistant to pull the cheek out to allow better vision in the mouth.

The timely use of a gum elastic bougie can make endotracheal intubation easier and less traumatic. The general principle of "a big cannula over a small guidewire" is widely used in medicine.

A size 8·0 mm endotracheal tube is used for adult females and 9·0 mm for adult males. This size refers to the *internal* diameter of the tube. Tubes are normally cut to a length of 21–23 cm.

Tracheostomy

Tracheostomy is used for airway control in the following circumstances:

- to bypass upper respiratory tract obstruction;
- for long-term ventilation;
- to facilitate suction of chest secretions;
- for prevention of aspiration of gastric contents (for example, bulbar palsy).

Conclusion

Obstruction of the airway must be prevented at all times—a patent airway is a happy airway.

3: Tracheal intubation

Tracheal intubation is an acquired skill. Hypoxia as a result of unrecognised oesophageal intubation can cause death.

Laryngoscopic views

The laryngoscopic views seen on intubation are often recorded by the anaesthetist and have been graded by Cormack and Lehane.

- Grade I   full view of glottis
- Grade II   only posterior commissure visible
- Grade III only tip of epiglottis visible
- Grade IV   no glottic structure visible.

Displacement

Tracheal tubes can be displaced after correct insertion. This is particularly likely when the patient is moved or the position changed. Flexion or extension of the head, or lateral neck movement, has been shown to cause movement of the tube of up to 5 cm within the trachea. Tracheal tubes should be fixed securely to minimise accidental extubation and the correct positioning should be checked regularly.

Confirmation of tracheal intubation

Confirmation is by clinical signs and technical tests. In the operating theatre both methods are used; however, elsewhere only clinical signs can be used.

Box 3.1   Clinical signs used to confirm tracheal intubation

- Direct visualisation of tracheal tube through vocal cords.
- Palpation of tube movement within the trachea.
- Chest movements.
- Breath sounds.
- Reservoir bag compliance and refill.
- Condensation of water vapour on clear tracheal tubes.

Direct visualisation of the tracheal tube passing through the vocal cords is the best clinical method of confirming tracheal intubation. This is normally achieved easily, but is not always possible in technically difficult intubations. All anaesthetists can recount situations where they *think* they have seen the tracheal tube pass through the vocal cords but subsequently found it in the oesophagus. Belief that the trachea is intubated can lead to a false sense of airway security if cyanosis occurs, and often other causes are sought for the hypoxaemia. The position of the tracheal tube must always be checked in these circumstances.

The other listed signs are helpful, but *unreliable*, in confirming correct placement of the tracheal tube.

Whilst an assistant applying cricoid pressure may "feel" the tube passing down the trachea, the same sensation can also occur with an oesophageal intubation. Observation of chest wall movement is no guarantee of correct tracheal tube placement. Movement is difficult to observe in some patients (obesity) and may also be seen in cases of oesophageal intubation.

Auscultation can be misleading: gas movement in the oesophagus can be transmitted to the lungs and so oesophageal sounds may be mistaken for lung sounds. Epigastric auscultation can be undertaken, but breath sounds again may be heard in the epigastrium, and so can cause confusion.

There is a characteristic "feel" to the breathing circuit reservoir bag which is often different when the oesophagus is intubated. Reservoir bag refilling will occur in tracheal intubation, but has been described after stomach distension with oesophageal intubation. A "rumbling" noise is often heard in oesophageal intubation which is distinct from that heard in tracheal intubation.

Condensation of water vapour is more likely to be seen with tracheal intubation, but can be present in gas emanating from the stomach and so is considered unreliable. If in doubt, and if at all possible, it is worth confirming correct tracheal tube placement by viewing again the tube passing through the larynx.

Technical tests

The commonly used tests are shown in Box 3.1.

> **Box 3.2   Technical tests to confirm intubation**
> - Negative pressure tests
> - End-tidal CO_2 monitoring–6 breaths
> - Fenum disposable CO_2 monitors
> - Fibreoptic observations of the trachea

Negative pressure tests rely on the fact that there are differences in the rigidity of the tracheal and oesophageal walls. Following intubation, a negative pressure is applied to the tube. Oesophageal walls are muscular and collapse upon application of a negative pressure and aspiration is prevented. Tracheal walls are rigid and, when a negative pressure is applied to the tube, tracheal gas can be aspirated. A negative pressure can be applied by using Wee's oesophageal detector device (Figure 3.1) which is a catheter mount attached to a 60 ml syringe.

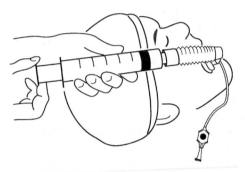

FIG 3.1—*An oesophageal detector*

An emptied, modified Ellick's evacuator bulb can also be attached to the tube and it will reinflate if in the trachea. False-positive results have been reported. It has been found to be impossible to aspirate a tracheal tube because of endobronchial intubation, or obstruction by the wall of the mucosa or by a mucous plug. The end-tidal CO_2 concentration can be measured using a capnograph. If pulmonary perfusion is adequate, end-tidal CO_2 concentration is about 5%. No CO_2 is excreted from the stomach, so any CO_2 present must be from the lungs. *Six breaths of CO_2* must be seen to confirm tracheal intubation. This is because alveolar CO_2 may have been ventilated into the upper gastrointestinal tract before intubation and it will take six breaths to excrete it from the stomach. Carbonated drinks may be present occasionally in the stomach and can cause some confusion. Fenum CO_2 analysers of disposable plastic contain a chemical indicator which changes colour on exposure to CO_2. These last several hours.

A fibreoptic laryngoscope placed through the endotracheal tube will show if tracheal placement is correct.

Although there are many tests to confirm tracheal intubation, the "gold standard" is six breaths of end-tidal CO_2 with visual confirmation of laryngeal placement of the tube.

Complications of tracheal intubation

(1) Laryngoscopy
- trauma to mouth, teeth, pharynx and larynx

- increased arterial pressure
- arrhythmias
- laryngospasm
- bronchospasm

(2) Immediate
  - oesophageal placement
  - pulmonary aspiration
  - displacement of tube from trachea
  - endobronchial intubation
  - airway obstruction: tube kinked, mucous plug, tracheal cuff herniation over lower end of tube

(3) Long-term
  - cord ulceration
  - tracheal stenosis
  - recurrent and superior laryngeal nerve damage.

The trainee needs to take special care to avoid the immediate complications. Tracheal tubes can easily kink, or be placed too far into the trachea and, either sit on the carina, or pass into the right main bronchus. High airway pressures may be seen when a patient is ventilated with these complications. Auscultation of the chest bilaterally may reveal a different intensity of breath sounds in endobronchial intubation. The tube is then pulled back and positioned correctly. Although almost invariably the tracheal tube passes into the right main bronchus, we have managed on rare occasions to intubate the left main bronchus.

Conclusion

The tracheal tube must be correctly sited and secured. Confirmation by direct observation of tracheal placement and six breaths of end-tidal CO_2 with continuous monitoring can avoid the potentially fatal consequences resulting from hypoxia. An anaesthetic maxim to remember when unsure of tracheal tube placement is:

IF IN DOUBT, TAKE IT OUT!

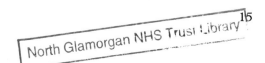

4: Failed intubation drill

It is essential to ask for assistance before anaesthetising patients who have been assessed as having potentially difficult airways. Failed tracheal intubation can occur in both elective and emergency anaesthesia. It is important to prepare a plan of management should intubation be impossible during the induction of general aneasthesia. We recommend that "failed intubation drills" be practised when accompanied by senior colleagues.

Initial strategy

The strategy for each case should be similar to that shown below. Calling for senior help, preventing hypoxia and not giving further doses of muscle relaxants when you are confronted by an impossible intubation are key points.

Box 4.1   Initial course of action for failed intubation

(1) *Plan* a course of management before starting anaesthesia.

(2) Call for *HELP.*
(3) Maintain airway.
(4) Ventilate with 100% oxygen.
(5) Maintain cricoid pressure (if part of anaesthetic technique).
(6) Avoid persistent attempts to intubate if patient is hypoxic.
(7) Avoid further doses of muscle relaxants unless you are absolutely sure of airway control and ventilation.

The airway must be patent and *oxygenation of the patient is mandatory.* Suxamethonium is the muscle relaxant with the fastest onset and is always used for emergency surgery, in patients with full stomachs, and in those who are at risk of regurgitation (for example, hiatus hernia). Experienced anaesthetists often use muscle relaxants of slower onset for elective surgical patients in whom they can be confident of airway control. Muscle relaxants should *not* be given inappropriately, for example in cases of upper airway obstruction. If a patient is paralysed, and tracheal intubation, patency of the upper airway, and oxygenation are impossible, then hypoxaemia and death will occur.

Secondary decisions

Once failed intubation has occurred, further decisions have to be made.

Box 4.2   Subsequent decisions for consideration after failed intubation

(1) Awaken patient or continue anaesthetic until senior help arrives.
(2) Summon experienced help—Intubate under general or local anaesthesia: laryngeal mask (intubation through mask), fibreoptic intubation, blind nasal intubation.
(3) Last resorts include retrograde intubation, transtracheal jet ventilation, cricothyroidotomy.
(4) Make elective tracheostomy.
(5) Perform surgery under regional anaesthesia.

The safest decision is to awaken the patient, although this may be modified by consideration of the elective or emergency nature of the surgery. Patients are not usually pleased to be woken up without undergoing surgery, but at least they are alive to complain! If airway control and ventilation are easy, or the patient reverts spontaneously to breathing in an unobstructed fashion and help is nearby, the anaesthetic may be continued. A laryngeal mask can secure airway patency when other methods have failed. Sometimes it is possible to continue the anaesthetic with the patient breathing spontaneously unintubated, but intubation may be mandatory.

Intubation can be achieved through a laryngeal mask airway, by blind nasal intubation techniques or via a fibreoptic laryngoscope. Rarely, retrograde intubation can be used. This technique involves cricothyroid membrane puncture and a guide catheter being pushed up through the larynx and out of the mouth. A tracheal tube can then be passed over the guiding catheter (the same principle as described in Chapter 3). Equipment for achieving airway control includes cricothyroid puncture devices which can be connected to a breathing circuit and transtracheal jet ventilation devices.

Formal tracheostomy may have to be considered. Abandonment of a general anaesthetic technique and implementation of surgery under regional analgesia is a sensible alternative.

After failed intubation, both the patient and other anaesthetists need to be informed of the difficulty in case of surgery at a later date.

(1) Note grade of intubation.
(2) Mark patient's notes boldly.
(3) Inform patient verbally and by letter.

The patient's folder containing the clinical records should be marked stating the anaesthetic problem.

Conclusion

Failed intubation should be prepared for and the priority initially should be on airway control and ventilation of the lungs. It is usually safer to awaken a patient and then consider the alternatives after consultation with a more experienced colleague.

A "failed intubation drill" should be committed to memory very early in the training programme and be practised at regular intervals. Sooner or later it will be needed.

5: Vascular access

Vascular access may be divided into venous (peripheral, central) and arterial. The novice anaesthetist will rapidly gain expertise in peripheral venous cannulation. We also think it important to become proficient in central venous cannulation and insertion of arterial cannulae, within the first few months of training. We have not included practical descriptions on how to undertake these procedures; these skills are best learnt by careful instruction from a senior anaesthetist.

Peripheral venous access

No general or regional anaesthetic procedure should start without intravenous access. A large bore cannula (14 or 16 gauge) or occasionally a small cannula (21 or 23 gauge) may be used, depending on the type of surgery. Flows through peripherally placed cannulae can be surprisingly high (Box 5.1). For any surgical procedure in which rapid blood loss may occur, nothing smaller than a 16 gauge cannula should be used. For major surgery at least one 14 gauge cannula is essential. The major determinant of the flow rate achieved through a cannula is the fourth power of the internal radius. All large bore intravenous cannulae, that are inserted before induction of anaesthesia, should be placed after the intradermal infiltration of lignocaine using a 25 gauge needle. The "sting" of the local anaesthetic is trivial compared with the pain of a large intravenous cannula pushed through the skin—we speak from bitter personal experience. Be kind to your patients.

Box 5.1 Flow rates through typical venous cannulae

Peripheral		Central	
Gauge	Flow (ml/min)	Gauge	Flow (ml/min)
23	16		
21	21		
18·5	48		
16	121	16	110
14	251	14	230

Central venous access

Central venous cannulation is undertaken to provide venous access when the peripheral route is unavailable, to measure central venous pressure, to administer drugs, and to provide parenteral nutrition.

There are two main routes by which anaesthetists acquire central venous access. Firstly, a long venous catheter may be inserted via the basilic vein in the antecubital fossa which will pass, one hopes, into the superior vena cava. The final position of the catheter needs confirmation by X-rays, as the catheter can pass up into the internal jugular vein and even down the other arm. There are few complications with this technique, although "damped" pressure recordings are often seen with long catheters, and enthusiastic insertion occasionally results in the measurement of right ventricular pressures!

Secondly, a technique involving cannulation of the internal jugular vein is used. The internal jugular vein arises as a continuation of the sigmoid sinus as it passes through the jugular foramen. It lies within the carotid sheath, lateral to the carotid artery and the vagus nerve, and runs beneath the sternal and clavicular heads of the sternomastoid muscle where it can be "palpated". It finally passes under the medial border of the clavicle to join the subclavian vein.

The right internal jugular vein is normally used as the veins are relatively straight on the right side of the neck and the thoracic duct is avoided. A strict aseptic technique with the patient in a head-down position is used. This fills the veins and avoids the risk of air embolism. A "high-neck" approach lessens the complications and the cannula can be inserted after ballotting the vein, or lateral to the carotid arterial pulsation. Some anaesthetists find it difficult to palpate the internal jugular vein, but it is often felt as the boggiest part of the neck lateral to the carotid artery. If the patient is hypovolaemic it can be impossible to ballotte the vein.

Although internal jugular vein cannulation is relatively safe in skilful hands, problems can occur (Box 5.2).

Box 5.2 Complications of internal jugular vein catheterisation

- Immediate
  - venous haematoma
  - carotid artery puncture haematoma
  - pneumothorax
  - haemothorax
  - nerve trauma (brachial plexus, vagus, phrenic)
  - air embolism

- Delayed
  - infection

Haematoma are the most common, and we have been impressed by the lack of problems following inadvertent carotid artery puncture. Pneumothorax should not occur with the "high-neck" approach. If you have more than 4 cm of the cannula inserted and still not found the vein, stop and try a different site.

Central venous pressure is measured from the midaxillary line via a pressure transducer or a water manometer. There is no normal central venous pressure. It is the response to an intravenous fluid load that determines whether the patient is hypovolaemic or not. The causes of variants in central venous pressure are shown in Box 5.3.

Box 5.3 Variants in central venous pressure

- Low pressure
  - hypovolaemia
  - respiratory phase variation

- High pressure
  - hypervolaemia
  - right ventricular dysfunction
  - increased right ventricular afterload
    - pulmonary hypertension
    - parenchymal pulmonary disease
    - pneumothorax
    - haemothorax
  - left heart failure
  - atrial arrhythmias
  - tricuspid valve disease

Arterial access

This is commonly performed via the radial artery with a 20 or 22 gauge cannula. An Allen's test may be done to assess the relative contributions of the radial and ulnar arteries to blood flow of the hand. This is done by occluding both the radial and ulnar arteries and then watching for "palmar flushing" when the ulnar artery is released. If flushing occurs, then it implies that, in the event of radial artery trauma or occlusion, the ulnar artery will supply the hand. In practice we never bother with Allen's test as its value is not proven. Complications of arterial cannulation include thrombosis, infection, fistula, aneurysm, and distal ischaemia. These are rare but, in the event of clinical ischaemia, the cannula should be removed and expert help sought urgently. Colour coding of arterial cannulae and their dedicated infusion tubing with red tags and red three-way taps should be undertaken if possible. This reduces the risk of inadvertent injection of drugs into arteries. We have seen the results of such accidents—gangrenous fingers are most unpleasant.

Conclusion

Intravenous access is mandatory before starting any form of anaesthesia, local or general. If there is *any* possibility of rapid blood loss, insert a large bore intravenous cannula. Lack of vascular access is a major contributor to anaesthetic disasters.

6: Intravenous fluids

Intravenous fluids and electrolytes are administered, often empirically, to replace or maintain the body's own requirements. Patients are starved preoperatively to ensure an empty stomach. There is much debate about how long a patient should be without fluids or food before elective surgery: 4–6 hours is often taken as the minimum requirement for food and 2–4 hours for clear fluids, but many patients starve overnight for at least 12 hours before anaesthesia.

Once you have inserted an intravenous cannula, it is necessary to give an appropriate fluid. The main choice is between crystalloid or colloid solutions. There are also glucose-containing solutions but it is difficult to make a case for continued use of such solutions. There is considerable debate about the relative merits of crystalloid or colloid solutions. In practice most anaesthetists start with 1–2 litres crystalloid and follow this with a similar volume of colloid solution in major surgery. Fluids are given intraoperatively to:

- replace existing deficits
- maintain fluid balance
- replace surgical loss.

The existing fluid deficit can be high, particularly with prolonged starvation in a warm environment; 1 litre of crystalloid given intravenously at the start of anaesthesia often only replaces an existing deficit. The rate of fluid administration is determined by assessing the adequacy of the circulating blood volume using the following indices:

- Arterial pressure
- Heart rate
- Central venous pressure (if available)
- Urine output
- Peripheral temperature (if available).

Crystalloids

Crystalloids are isotonic solutions which have a similar fluid and electrolyte composition to the extracellular fluid. These solutions are confined to the extracellular space in a ratio of 1:3 in terms of intravascular: interstitial volume. The two commonly available solutions are Hartmann's solution and 0·9% sodium chloride solution. The lactate in Hartmann's solution is either oxidised in the liver, or undergoes gluconeogenesis. Both metabolic pathways use hydrogen ions so that mild alkalinisation occurs. It is important to remember that both these solutions add little to the intravascular volume.

Glucose-containing solutions

It is difficult to make a case for continuing to use these solutions. The stress of surgery increases circulating blood glucose so that the addition of more glucose intravenously exacerbates the metabolic insult. Furthermore, when glucose is eventually oxidised to water and carbon dioxide, the infusion is then equivalent to water only (5% glucose) or a very weak hypotonic solution (4% glucose + 0·18% sodium chloride solution). The main reason for continuing to use these solutions seems to be fear of the phase of sodium retention that inevitably accompanies surgery. Since *low* plasma sodium concentrations are almost invariably found postoperatively, this fear is unsubstantiated—patients usually need more sodium. Only a small proportion of glucose-containing solutions stay within the intravascular space; they are of little value in maintaining the blood volume. The composition of commonly used intravenous fluids is shown in Box 6.1.

Colloids

These are large molecules suspended in solution. They generate a colloid osmotic pressure and are confined to the intravascular space. They rarely cause allergic reactions as a side effect. Elimination is via the kidneys. There are two main types in clinical practice:

- Modified gelatins
- Hydroxyethyl starch.

The modified gelatins are "Haemaccel" (polygeline) and "Gelofusine" (succinylated gelatin). The electrolytic composition and properties are shown in Boxes 6.1 and 6.2, respectively, the properties being compared with albumin.

Box 6.1 Electrolytic composition of intravenous solutions (mmol/l)

Solution	Na	K	Ca	Cl	Lactate
0·9% Sodium chloride	150	—	—	150	—
Hartmann's solution	131	5	2	111	29
5% Glucose	—	—	—	—	—
4% Glucose in 0·18% NaCl	30	—	—	30	—
Gelofusine	154	—	—	125	—
Haemaccel	145	5	6	145	—
Hydroxyethyl starch	154	—	—	154	—

Box 6.2 Properties of colloid solutions

	M.W.	Plasma $t_{1/2}$ (h)	Elimination	Anaphylaxis
Albumin	69 000	24	slow	nil
Haemaccel	35 000	3	rapid	rare
Gelofusine	30 000	3	rapid	rare
Hydroxyethyl starch	450 000	6–9	slow	rare

Haemaccel contains calcium which can cause clotting in an intravenous infusion set when it becomes mixed with citrated blood and plasma.

Hydroxyethyl starch is taken up by the reticuloendothelial system after phagocytosis in the blood, and this results in its prolonged degradation and elimination. The maximum dose is limited to 20 ml/kg/day.

Conclusion

Fluid therapy is simple. Start with 1–2 litres crystalloid solution (Hartmann's solution or 0·9% sodium chloride) and follow this, if necessary, with a suitable colloid solution. Do not use glucose-containing solutions without a good reason and, if there is marked blood loss, consider red cell replacement (Chapter 12).

7: The anaesthetic machine

The anaesthetic machine delivers known gas and vapour concentrations which are variable in amount and composition. The machine is of a "continuous-flow" nature and designed so that gases are administered at safe pressures.

The machine has six basic components (Box 7.1).

Box 7.1   Anaesthetic machine components

- Gas supply—cylinders, pipelines and pressure gauges
- Pressure regulators
- Flow meter needle valves
- Rotameters
- Vaporisers
- Common gas outlet

Anaesthetic machines vary in age, and the different nomenclature for pressure readings can cause confusion. The derived (Système Internationale) SI unit of pressure is the pascal and pressure in the anaesthetic machine is measured in kilopascals (kPa). The comparative factors for other units of pressure are shown in Box 7.2.

Box 7.2   One atmosphere of pressure (various units)

- 760 mm Hg
- 1034 cm H_2O
- 15 lb/in^2
- 101 kPa
- 1 bar

Gas supply

Cylinders

These are made of molybdenum steel and are colour-coded:

- N_2O: blue body, blue shoulder
- O_2:   black body, white shoulder
- CO_2:   grey body, grey shoulder
- Air: grey body, white/black shoulder.

To prevent incorrect placement of the cylinder onto the machine, a pin-index system has been devised. On each cylinder is an arrangement of three holes specific to the gas and there is a corresponding pin on the machine. A washer (Bodok seal) is necessary on the top pin to stop leaks occurring between the cylinder and the machine.

An oxygen cylinder contains gas and the pressure in a full cylinder is $137 \times 100\,kPa$. The pressure decreases linearly as the cylinder empties. Nitrous oxide is a liquified gas at a pressure of $52 \times 100\,kPa$. The pressure in the cylinder remains the same as it empties, until all the liquid becomes gaseous (when cylinder is about a quarter full) and only then does the pressure start to drop.

Pipelines

Pipelines from a central supply can be connected directly to the machine. These are again colour coded:

- O_2: white
- N_2O: blue
- suction pipeline: yellow.

They are made of copper and outlets from the pipeline system are identified by name, colour, and shape. They have noninterchangeable Schrader valve connections.

Oxygen normally comes from a liquid cryogenic source and nitrous oxide from central banks of cylinders. The pressure of pipeline supplied gases is $4 \times 100\,kPa$.

Pressure regulators

Beneath the machine are pressure-reducing valves (Figure 7.1) which regulate the pressure entering the machine. Gas at high pressure enters and passes through a small port to a low pressure chamber. As the pressure here rises, the diaphragm is pushed up against the spring and the valve is closed. If the outlet valve is opened, the pressure drops and the spring will push the diaphragm down, and the whole process starts again. Pressure of all gases now entering the machine is 4×100 kPa.

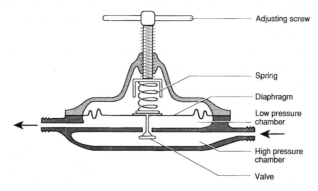

FIG 7.1—*A pressure-reducing valve*

Flow meter needle valve

The pressure is about atmospheric at the common gas outlet of the machine and the main pressure drop from 4×100 kPa occurs across the needle valve at the base of the rotameters (Figure 7.2).

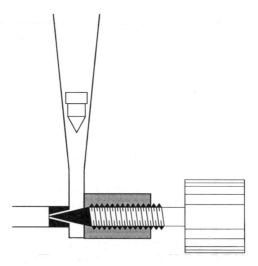

FIG 7.2—*Flow meter needle valve and rotameter*

The knobs are colour-coded; the oxygen knob is bigger than the others and of a wider, grooved nature. This enables it to be identified in darkness. In the United Kingdom it is the convention for the oxygen valve to be mounted on the left side of the machine.

Rotameters

These are calibrated specifically for each gas and are noninterchangeable. Cracks in the rotameter tubing may lead to hypoxic mixtures being produced, so an oxygen gas analyser is positioned at the common gas outlet on the machine.

The scale on the rotameter is nonlinear as the rotameters themselves are tapered. Low gas flows, when using carbon dioxide absorption circuits, need to be very accurate.

Vaporisers

These convert a volatile liquid anaesthetic to a continuous flow anaesthetic vapour mixed with gases, under controlled conditions. Thermal energy is used in converting a liquid to a vapour and a temperature drop occurs within the liquid. Variable rates of vaporisation will occur unless this is compensated for. Temperature compensation (Tec-type) vaporisers are in common use and compensation is achieved by means of a bimetallic strip within the machine.

A vaporiser should be constructed of materials of high specific heat and high thermal conductivity. Copper is used, although this is not ideal, and within the vaporiser are a series of copper helical wicks which provide a large surface area, ensuring that a saturated vapour pressure exists within the machine at all times.

Vaporisers should be filled at the end of the operating list to decrease pollution. There is a noninterchangeable filling device which ensures that the vaporiser is filled with the correct agent. Vaporisers are connected to the "back bar" of the anaesthetic machine and an "O" ring washer system must be present at this site to stop leaks.

Common gas outlet

The gases finally pass from the machine via the common gas outlet at about atmospheric pressure. The oxygen analyser is connected here.

In addition to the Bourdon-type pressure gauges which measure the cylinder and pipeline pressure, three other features on the machine must be noted.

- Oxygen flush. This button delivers oxygen at a rate of 30 l/min to the common gas outlet, bypassing the vaporisers and flowmeters.
- Hypoxic or oxygen failure alarm. This device causes the nitrous oxide to be cut or dumped if the oxygen supply is <21%. This can occur if the oxygen rotameter is accidentally bumped or turned down. An audible alarm is heard when this is activated.
- Pressure relief valve. On the "back bar" between the common gas outlet and the vaporisers, there is a pressure release valve which protects the

machine against excessive pressure caused by obstruction to gas flow beyond the common gas outlet. This does not protect the patient but is designed to protect the machine. It is activated by back pressure in excess of a third of an atmosphere (35 kPa).

Checking the anaesthetic machine

Absolute familiarity with the anaesthetic machine is fundamental for safe practice. It *must* be checked before an operating list and six items need inspection (Box 7.3).

> ### Box 7.3   Anaesthetic machine checklist
> - Oxygen analyser
> - Gas supply
> - Vaporisers
> - Breathing systems
> - Ventilator
> - Suction apparatus and other checks

Oxygen analyser

This fuel cell is normally calibrated by a single point calibration to room air—21%. The sensor should then be attached firmly to the common gas outlet.

Gas supply

This is done to ensure that the correct gas supplies and connections exist within the machine, to check pressures and to stop the accidental delivery of a hypoxic gas mixture. These checks, with familiarity, take about five minutes and involve seven steps.

- *Step 1*
  - Disconnect machine from the pipelines.
  - Remove the carbon dioxide and other unwanted cylinders.
  - The oxygen and nitrous oxide cylinders should be sealed correctly and turned "off".
  - "Blank" empty yokes.
  - Vaporisers "off".
  - ALL flowmeters should be opened.

- *Step 2*
  - Turn *oxygen* cylinder fully "on".
  - Adjust oxygen flow rate on rotameter to 5 l/min.

- Check pressure gauge—full cylinder 137×100 kPa.
- Oxygen analyser should read 100%.

- *Step 3*
  - Turn *nitrous oxide* cylinder fully "on".
  - Set nitrous oxide flow rate on rotameter to 5 l/min.
  - Check pressure gauge—pressure reads 52×100 kPa (remember pressure remains constant until cylinder is only quarter full).

- *Step 4*
  - Turn *oxygen* cylinder "off".
  - Press oxygen bypass (pipelines empty of oxygen).
  - Oxygen cylinder pressure returns to zero.
  - ALARM sounds (oxygen protection device) and nitrous oxide is dumped or cut.

- *Step 5*
  - Connect oxygen pipeline to central supply.
  - "Tug" test—pull connection to ensure it is not loose.
  - Oxygen failure protection device is cancelled.
  - Oxygen flow is restored.
  - Pipeline pressure gauge will read 4×100 kPa.

- *Step 6*
  - Turn nitrous oxide cylinder "off".
  - Connect nitrous oxide pipeline to central supply.
  - "Tug" test.
  - Nitrous oxide flow is restored.
  - Pipeline pressure gauge will read 4×100 kPa.

- *Step 7*
  - Check other cylinders (if any).
  - Turn "off" oxygen flowmeter.
  - Check that any antihypoxic device will reduce nitrous oxide flow.
  - Turn "off" ALL flowmeters.
  - Press oxygen flush; check there is no decrease in pipeline pressure and O_2 analyser shows 100%.

Vaporisers

- Check "O" rings present on back bar.
- Check for correct mounting and filling.
- Turn "on"—check for leaks—turn "off"—recheck for leaks (check for leaks by occluding common gas outlet after opening oxygen rotameter to a 5 l/min flow).

31

Breathing systems

- Check the configuration of the system.
- Check for leaks in the reservoir bag and that expiratory valve does not stick.
- Check for leaks in the circuit.
- Check tightness of all connections (push and twist technique).

Ventilator

- Check for familiarity of ventilator.
- Check configuration.
- Check operation.
- Check alarm system works and set alarm limits.
- Set controls.

Suction apparatus and other checks

- Check suction works (maximum pressure for suction is 80 kPa).
- Check table tilts.
- Check for at least two working laryngoscopes, and correctly sized tracheal tubes and intubating aids.
- Check tracheal tube cuffs.
- Check monitoring equipment present, switch on and set alarms.

Conclusion

The novice anaesthetist must have a thorough knowledge of the basic workings of an anaesthetic machine and checking the machine must become a regular habit. The start of work in operating theatres should be signalled by a cacophony of alarms, as all the machines are checked before use. Do not assume, however, that, because the machine was checked early in the morning, nothing can go wrong for the rest of the day. Machines are moved and knocked, pipelines stretched and vaporisers changed. *Remain vigilant.*

8: Anaesthetic breathing systems

Anaesthetic breathing systems are classified into three main groups (Box 8.1).

Box 8.1   Classification of breathing systems

- Systems using carbon dioxide absorption
- Rebreathing systems
- Non-rebreathing systems

Components

Each circuit consists of a variable number of components and is often made as a single unit, rather than needing to be assembled from individual items (Box 8.2).

Box 8.2   Anaesthetic breathing circuit components

- Breathing hoses
- Bags
- Adjustable pressure-limiting valves (APL)
- Connections
- Carbon dioxide absorption
- Unidirectional valves.

Breathing hoses

These are corrugated 22 mm diameter plastic or rubber tubes which are nonkinkable and noncompliant. They have a volume of 400–450 ml/m, and the newer plastic hoses are more prone to pin-hole leaks than older rubber hoses, so circuits must be checked.

Bags

These are made of rubber and are of 2 litre volume in adult circuits and 500 ml volume in paediatric circuits. They have four functions (Box 8.3).

> ## Box 8.3   Functions of bags in breathing systems
>
> - Reservoir for gases. Although the machine can deliver flow rates of up to 10–20 l/min of gas, the patient has brief inspiratory flow rates of up to 30 l/min. To facilitate the delivery of this high flow rate, a reservoir of gas must exist.
> - Monitoring of respiration.
> - Facilitating manual intermittent positive pressure ventilation.
> - Pressure limiting function. The bag can distend to large volumes without pressure within the system increasing greatly. This safety feature avoids barotrauma to the patient's lungs if the pressure-limiting valve malfunctions or is omitted from the circuit.

Adjustable pressure-limiting valves (APL)

These variable orifice, variable resistance devices vent excess gases. They often have a scavenging facility. They consist of a light disc held onto a circular knife edge by a light spring with tension. The spring is adjusted by a screw thread.

When the valve is set fully open, the pressure to open the disc and hence the valve, is only 0·1–0·2 kPa (1–2 cm H_2O), and minimal resistance to flow occurs. When the valve is closed, a safety device protects the patient by opening at a pressure of about 6 kPa (60 cm H_2O). This occurs at a gas flow of 30 l/min.

Connections

Connections are achieved by 22 mm or 15 mm male to female fittings.

Carbon dioxide absorption

Sodalime is used for this. It contains 80% calcium hydroxide, 4% sodium hydroxide, 1% potassium hydroxide and the remainder is water. It contains an indicator which changes colour as the mixture is exhausted, and a hardener which is silica gel.

Absorption occurs via the following chemical reaction:

$$CO_2 + H_2O \rightarrow H_2CO_3$$

$$H_2CO_3 + 2NaOH \rightarrow Na_2CO_3 + 2H_2O$$

$$Na_2CO_3 + Ca(OH)_2 \rightarrow CaCO_3 + 2NaOH$$

Potassium hydroxide behaves similarly to sodium hydroxide. Heat is produced in this reaction. Small amounts of gases and vapours are also absorbed.

Unidirectional valves

These ensure one-way flow in circle systems.

Systems using carbon dioxide absorption

The circle system employs unidirectional valves to direct gas flow through hoses, a reservoir bag, and sodalime. Oxygen and the volatile vapour are added. As the inspired gases are free of carbon dioxide, the patient can rebreathe without adverse physiological effects. Low gas flows can be used and the rotameters must be accurate.

The system is economical, conserves heat and moisture, and decreases pollution. However, to be efficient it must be free from leaks. Oxygen, carbon dioxide, and anaesthetic vapour analysis is mandatory. Dilution of gases in the reservoir bag by nitrogen in the early part of the anaesthetic can occur—higher gas flows in the first five minutes are recommended.

Oxygen uptake from the lungs is relatively constant at 200–250 ml/min, but nitrous oxide uptake is high initially (500 ml/min), falling to 200 ml/min after half an hour, and 100 ml/min after 60 minutes. Therefore, hypoxic mixtures are possible at low flows and this is one reason why an oxygen analyser must be incorporated in the system.

The position of the vaporiser in the circuit is important. It is usually outside the circle (VOC) when conventional vaporisers can be used. However, occasionally it is placed within the circle (VIC) and then must be of low resistance.

Rebreathing systems

Traditionally these systems have no separation of the inspired and expired gases, although in the newer coaxial systems partition of the gases occurs. Under conditions of low fresh gas flow or hyperventilation of the patient, rebreathing of carbon dioxide is possible. Flow rates of gases should be adjusted according to capnography. Classification of rebreathing systems was first described by Mapleson in 1954. There are six basic systems (Figure 8.1) and two involving a coaxial arrangement (Figure 8.2).

The *Mapleson A* is also called the Magill attachment. Fresh gas flow should equal alveolar minute ventilation for spontaneous respiration and be 2–2·5 times the alveolar minute ventilation for intermittent positive pressure ventilation. This is the most efficient system for spontaneously breathing patients and the least efficient for intermittent positive pressure ventilation. The system is heavy with the valve in its traditional position and access is often difficult; because of this it was modified by Lack to

35

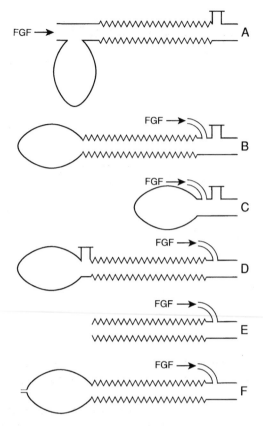

FIG 8.1—*Mapleson classification of rebreathing systems. Arrows indicate direction of fresh gas flow (FGF)*

incorporate a coaxial system where the valve was at the machine end of the circuit. In the Lack circuit, inspiration is through a large outer tube and expiration takes place through a smaller inner tube of low resistance.

The *Mapleson B and C* circuits are used infrequently, but the C is useful for brief periods of manual ventilation.

The *Mapleson D, E and F* systems are T-pieces at the patient end of the circuit and differ only in the way they vent the gases. The Mapleson D is the most efficient for intermittent positive pressure ventilation.

The *Bain* circuit is a coaxial Mapleson D with a 22 mm diameter outer tube and 7 mm diameter inner tube. The gases enter via the inner tube. It is light, often disposable, has the gas entry and the expiratory valve at the machine end, and has a clear outer tube to ensure that the inner tube can be seen to be attached and not kinked. Leaks or holes in the inner tubing cause rapid carbon dioxide rebreathing. To check that there are no leaks in the inner tube, it should be occluded (fifth finger or 2 ml syringe). Oxygen flows of 5 l/min into the system will cause the anaesthetic machine

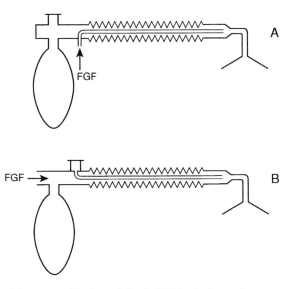

FIG 8.2—*Coaxial systems of Bain and Lack. FGF=fresh gas flow*

back-bar pressure-releasing alarm to blow as the occlusion pressure is transmitted along the machine. The reservoir bag should *not* distend.

Flow rates using this system are high, at least 70–100 ml/kg/min and up to two to three times the minute alveolar ventilation are recommended, but should be adjusted according to capnography.

The *Mapleson E and F* systems incorporate the Ayre's T-piece, have no adjustable pressure limiting valves, and are used for children under 20–25 kg, again at flows of two to three times the minute alveolar ventilation. The open-ended reservoir bag of the Jackson–Rees modification (Mapleson F) was added to assist intermittent positive pressure ventilation rather than occluding the end of the Mapleson E system, although spontaneous ventilation can be monitored by its movement.

Non-rebreathing systems

These use one-way, or non-rebreathing, valves to direct and separate the inspired and expired gases. They are not used in the operating theatre, but are seen in the "draw-over" system for field anaesthesia where compressed gases are unavailable (Triservice devices). They are low resistance systems, as the patient's inspiratory efforts cause gas flow and a low resistance draw-over vaporiser must be used. Inflating bellows can be added for ventilation purposes.

Conclusion

Anaesthetic breathing circuits may appear confusing initially, but the principles are simple. Modern monitoring facilities, particularly capnography and oxygen analysis, enable appropriate fresh gas flows to be used whatever circuit is employed. The breathing circuits are the most common site for gas leaks. *Check carefully.*

9: Ventilators and other equipment

Ventilators

Ventilation can be delivered to the lung by two methods:

- Negative pressure devices. A negative pressure is applied externally around the thorax (cuirass ventilators).
- Positive pressure devices. A positive pressure is applied to the lungs via the trachea. This is the method used in theatre and these devices are driven by one of three methods: gas, electricity, separate supply of compressed air or oxygen.

There are five types of ventilators (Box 9.1).

> ### Box 9.1 Ventilator types
>
> - Mechanical thumbs
> - Minute volume dividers
> - Bag squeezers
> - Intermittent flow generators
> - High frequency ventilators

Mechanical thumbs are only used with T-piece circuits. Bag squeezers are widely used with circle systems where a pneumatic bellows device operates intermittently.

Intermittent flow generators have a control mechanism which interrupts intermittently a flow of gas from a high pressure source (for example, a cylinder). These can be made compact and are used for ventilation during transportation. High frequency ventilators deliver very small tidal volumes at very high rates to maintain normal gas exchange.

A typical example of a minute volume divider is the Manley ventilator. This ventilator is powered by the pressure of the gases from the anaesthetic machine. The minute volume is determined by the volume setting on the flow meters and this gas distends weight-loaded bellows. Gas flow to and from the patient is controlled by two linked valves. Inspiration occurs by opening of the inspiratory valve and closure of the expiratory valve. In expiration the reverse occurs. This simple, cheap device does not allow rebreathing to occur, can be scavenged, and contains a manual mode reservoir breathing bag.

The machine requires the following functions to be set:

- Two switches must be set to operate the ventilator in manual or ventilator mode.
- The tidal volume must be set.
- The pressure of the weight-loaded bellows must be set.
- The time of the inspiratory phase must be set.

The ventilator is far from ideal. It is a pressure-generated ventilator and the flow from the ventilator is affected by patient characteristics. In bronchospasm, for example, it will not function correctly. Ideally the volume delivered by a ventilator should not change in response to alterations in respiratory compliance. Flow-generated ventilators, which are often used in intensive care units, meet this requirement.

Never use a ventilator unless you have received clear instructions about how it functions. Most patients anaesthetised in theatre require only simple ventilators and the trend towards increasing complexity is to be deplored. We have seen recently a ventilator that had over thirty possible settings. Although it may be of value in intensive care, in theatre it is a disaster waiting to happen. The ideal ventilator has no more than three knobs!

Whenever the lungs are ventilated it is *imperative* that the following monitoring is available:

- disconnection alarm
- expired minute volume
- capnography
- inspired oxygen concentration beyond the ventilator
- airway pressure.

Other monitoring may be used, as required. However, the basic monitoring ensures that the circuit is intact without leaks and that ventilation is adequate with a suitable inspired oxygen concentration.

Suction devices (Box 9.2)

These consist of three basic components.

Box 9.2 Suction device components

- Vacuum generating pump. This is normally located centrally within the hospital. The yellow piping in theatre is noninterchangeable and the suction system is connected to a high displacement pump that is linked by a series of anticontamination traps to a central reservoir.
- Reservoir in theatre to contain the fluid aspirated. A filter with a float mechanism exists within the reservoir to stop contamination of the pump by aspirated fluid.
- Delivery tubing which is disposable and is connected to flexible or rigid (Yankauer) catheters. Prolonged endotracheal suction can cause lung collapse and bradycardia, and should not be used.

The acceptable flow rate for suction devices is 35 l/min of air at a maximum of 80 kPa negative pressure.

Scavenging apparatus

Chronic and short-term exposure to inhalational anaesthetic agents is considered to be detrimental to the health of theatre workers, although conclusive evidence of impaired concentration, physical health, and fetal well-being in pregnant women is not proven.

On balance it seems sensible to scavenge waste gases. Scavenging systems consist of three components (Box 9.3).

Box 9.3 Scavenging system components

- Collecting system. This is a shroud enclosing the APL valve of the breathing system. The connection is of 30 mm diameter to prevent accidental connection to the breathing system circuit (22 mm).

- Receiving system. This has a reservoir to ensure adequate removal of gases. A rubber bag, or a rigid bottle, is often used and this ensures that removal of gases occurs even if the volume cleared is less than the peak expiratory flow rate.

- Disposal system. Three systems are used to remove the gases:
  - Passive. Through wide-bore tubing to a terminal ventilator in the roof. Disposal is dependent on wind direction.
  - Assisted passive. The air-conditioning system extractor ducts remove the gases.
  - Active. A dedicated ejector flowmeter or fan system is used. A low pressure, high volume system able to remove 75 l/min (with a peak flow of 130 l/min) is used.

Humidification

Humidification of inspired air occurs in the nose and naso/oropharynx. It is saturated by the time it reaches the trachea. Delivery of dry gases to the trachea by tracheal tubes can cause decreased ciliary activity, tenacious mucus, and even atelectasis.

In the operating theatre, humidification is usually carried out by a passive method using a "heat and moisture exchanger" filter. The filter is connected between the breathing circuit and the laryngeal mask or endotracheal tube. A hydrophobic membrane within the filter acts to retain water vapour and heat, and helps maintain the humidity of the anaesthetic gases in the patient's respiratory tract. The filter is disposable, has a low resistance to gas flow and removes bacteria and viruses. It prevents contamination of the breathing circuit and must be changed after every patient.

10: Monitoring in anaesthesia

An important source of anaesthetic-related morbidity and mortality remains human error. All anaesthetists have tales of "near-misses"; those anaesthetists who claim never to have problems are either doing insufficient work or are economical with the truth. A critical incident register is recommended in every anaesthetic department. A critical incident is an untoward event which, if left uncorrected, would have led to anaesthetic-related mortality or morbidity. It includes many events ranging from disconnection of the breathing circuit to unrecognised oesophageal intubation and severe bronchospasm. It is hoped that better monitoring will reduce the incidence of these complications.

Appropriate monitoring must occur wherever anaesthesia is conducted, whether it is in the anaesthetic room, the operating theatre, the psychiatric department, the X-ray department, or in dental surgeries.

Indeed, anaesthetising "away from home" outside the operating theatres demands particular care and appropriate monitoring *must be present.*

Monitoring facilities have improved greatly in recent years but still fall short of two of the requirements of anaesthesia:

- the ability to monitor cerebral oxygenation;
- the ability to monitor routinely the depth of anaesthesia.

Full monitoring has three requirements (Box 10.1).

Box 10.1   Anaesthesia monitoring requirements

- Presence of anaesthetist

- Checking and monitoring anaesthetic equipment

- Patient monitoring
  - clinical
  - technical

Anaesthetist

The anaesthetist *must* be present throughout the whole surgical procedure and be readily available to recovery room staff until the patient leaves the theatre complex. *This responsibility is solely the anaesthetist's*, and is applicable in general and regional anaesthesia, and also in some sedation techniques where the anaesthetist is involved.

An adequate record must be made of the whole anaesthetic process, from the induction to full recovery of the patient. Errors can occur for a variety of reasons ranging from inexperience and lack of training to tiredness, boredom, and inattention. Vigilance in an anaesthetist is a function of self-motivation.

The novice anaesthetist should acquire rigorous monitoring habits. Tracheal intubation must be confirmed *every* time and the equipment, the anaesthetic machine and circuitry checked as a routine. Postoperative visits to assess a patient's progress are salutary and give an opportunity to improve aspects of care such as postoperative analgesia, nausea, and vomiting.

Checking and monitoring equipment

Checking and monitoring the function of anaesthetic equipment has already been discussed in preceding chapters. The means of maintaining airway control, intravenous fluids and infusion devices must be understood, the anaesthetic machine, circuits and ventilators must be checked. Two key features must be emphasised—the oxygen supply and the breathing systems.

Oxygen supply

The gas supply to the oxygen flowmeter must contain a low pressure warning device and have an audible alarm.

If hypoxic mixtures can be delivered (most old machines), then a device which monitors continuously the concentration of oxygen delivered to the patient must be fitted and have an audible alarm.

Breathing system

If faults exist in the circuit, these are best detected by monitoring the expired volume, the end-tidal carbon dioxide concentration and by measuring the airway pressure (high pressure alarm). Clinical observation of the reservoir bag may reveal leaks, disconnections, and overdistension from high pressure. During mechanical ventilation measurement of the airway pressure, the expired volume, and carbon dioxide concentration are mandatory (see Chapter 9).

The alarm limits for equipment should be reset for each case and alarms should be turned ON (not turned off because the limits are being exceeded for a particular patient, but are not causing concern).

Patient monitoring

Clinical

The continuous observation of the patient's colour, chest movement and pattern of respiration, absence or presence of sweating and lacrimation, reactions of the pupil, use of a stethoscope, and palpation of a peripheral pulse provide essential basic monitoring of the patient. Much useful information can be obtained by simple observation, palpation, and auscultation—arts that are rapidly disappearing from anaesthesia.

Technical

The circulation and ventilation need continuous monitoring in all forms of anaesthesia. If muscle relaxants are used, a peripheral nerve stimulator should be used. The devices used routinely are shown in Box 10.2.

Box 10.2   Patient monitoring devices

- Cardiovascular
  - heart rate
  - electrocardiogram
  - noninvasive arterial pressure
  - oximeter

- Respiration
  - respiratory rate
  - end-tidal carbon dioxide concentration
  - inspired oxygen

- Muscle relaxation
  - peripheral nerve stimulator

In specialised surgery, facilities for further monitoring are required (Box 10.3).

Box 10.3   Specialised patient monitoring devices

- Invasive arterial pressure
- Central venous pressure
- Pulmonary artery pressure
- Concentration of volatile anaesthetic agent
- Urine output
- Temperature measurement
- Measurement of blood loss
- Biochemical analysis: pH, arterial gas analysis, electrolytes
- Haematological analysis: haemoglobin, coagulation studies

The *electrocardiogram* needs special emphasis because it is important to remember that electrical activity can exist even though there is no adequate cardiac output. Its value lies principally in monitoring changes in heart rate and in the diagnosis of arrhythmias.

Oximetry depends upon the differing absorption of light at different wavelengths by the various states of haemoglobin. Oxyhaemoglobin and reduced haemoglobin differ at both the red and infrared portions of the spectrum. The absorption is the same at 805 nm, the isobestic point. A pulse oximeter has two light sources on one side of the probe and a photodiode which generates a voltage when light falls upon it. The two emitting light sources are at 660 nm red (visible), and at 800 nm infrared (not visible).

The tissues absorb light but enough is transmitted to reach the photodiode. The arrival of the arteriolar pulsation with oxygenated blood alters the amount of red and infrared light transmitted through to the finger. This change is calculated by a microprocessor and the amount of oxygenated blood in the tissue deduced.

The sigmoid shape of the oxygen dissociation curve means that saturations of above 90% show adequate tissue oxygenation.

Oximetry is unreliable in the following instances:

- excessive movement
- venous congestion
- excessive illumination
- nail polish/false nails
- intravenous drugs: methylene blue, indocyanine green
- carbon monoxide poisoning.

The size and the shape of the arteriolar pulsation is shown as a plethysmographic trace.

Capnography is used to measure carbon dioxide. This utilises the principle of infrared absorption. When infrared light falls on a molecule, it enhances the molecule's vibrational energy and the infrared light is absorbed by the molecule. The amount of infrared light absorbed at a specific wavelength is proportional to the amount of carbon dioxide present in the gas mixture.

In the presence of a stable cardiac output, arterial carbon dioxide tension is related inversely to alveolar ventilation.

$$P_aCO_2 \; \alpha \; 1/V_A$$

Common causes of high and low P_aCO_2 are shown in Box 10.4.

Full monitoring equipment should be available in the recovery room, as well as in theatre. It must also be available for the transportation and transfer of patients.

46

Box 10.4   Common causes of high and low P_aCO_2

- Low
  - hyperventilation
  - low cardiac output: embolism (gas or blood)
- High
  - hypoventilation
  - rebreathing carbon dioxide: circuit failures
  - hypermetabolic states: malignant hyperthermia

Conclusion

The most important monitor during any anaesthetic procedure is the presence of a trained, vigilant anaesthetist. *Under no circumstances must you ever leave the theatre while a patient is under your care.*

Careful, repetitive clinical observation of the patient is the next essential procedure, followed by the appropriate use of monitors to assess the respiratory and cardiovascular system.

These principles apply to all surgical procedures. There are "small operations", but there is no such thing as a "small anaesthetic".

Part II
Crises and complications

As soon as you are capable of assessing and controlling the airway, ventilating the lungs and establishing vascular access, it is likely that you will be given a bleep. As the "on-call" anaesthetist, your problems have now started, as you will be expected to assess and start the management of a large number of anaesthetic problems around the hospital. In this section of the book we describe a variety of crises and complications. Some are common, such as cardiac arrest and massive haemorrhage, whereas others, such as malignant hyperthermia, are rare. Unfortunately, patients cannot be relied on to respect your lack of experience and they have the uncanny habit of keeping the most unusual complications for the most junior members of staff at the most unsocial hours.

11: Cardiac arrest

It is imperative that you have a detailed knowledge of the management of cardiac arrest. In the operating theatre, and often on the wards, you will be responsible for making the decisions. The causes of cardiac arrest are broadly classified as follows:

- medical diseases;
- surgical causes, especially haemorrhage (occult or massive) and occasionally vagal responses to surgical traction;
- anaesthetic causes, especially hypoxia and hypercapnia from problems such as failure to secure the airway and ventilate the lungs and unnoticed disconnection of the anaesthetic circuit; also from technical disasters such as a tension pneumothorax after attempts at central venous cannulation.

Endotracheal intubation

The endotracheal tube must be correctly positioned and secured. When there is no cardiac output, no carbon dioxide is produced; the capnograph (which is normally not available in the ward) is thus valueless in assessing correct positioning of the tracheal tube. Visualisation of the tube passing through the laryngeal opening is critically important and auscultation is used to ensure it is placed in the trachea and not the bronchus.

The capnograph may be a guide to the adequacy of the cardiac output when cardiopulmonary resuscitation is undertaken.

Defibrillation

Whenever you start to work in a new environment you *must* know where the defibrillator is kept and how it works. It should be tested every day without fail. A defibrillator is a capacitor and thus stores electrical charge. Usually it has four controls: on, charge, defibrillate, and synchronisation.

Oxygenation

It is essential that the lungs are ventilated with 100% oxygen. An oxygen analyser should be attached to the anaesthetic machine to confirm the nature of the fresh gas flow. (Check that the vaporisers are turned off.) If doubt exists, oxygen from a cylinder can be used.

Obstetrics

Fortunately pregnant patients very rarely suffer from a cardiac arrest. If they do, you will see a severe case of "obstetrician's distress"—an awesome sight. If the woman is <25 weeks pregnant, she can be treated as a nonpregnant adult. If she is >25 weeks pregnant, then there are two priorities. Firstly, the baby should be delivered immediately. Secondly, resuscitation must *not* occur with the patient in the supine position. The uterus will compress the inferior vena cava and inadequate venous return to the heart will result, with subsequent failure of patient resuscitation. Cardiopulmonary resuscitation should be made with the woman in a left lateral tilt to diminish caval compression. This can be achieved by a physical wedge, or by table tilt. A human wedge can be made by a member of the team kneeling on the floor and subsequently sitting on their heels. The woman is then positioned so that her back is on the thighs of the human wedge. Pregnant patients can be more difficult to intubate than nonpregnant women.

Adult resuscitation

Several Resuscitation Councils have issued guidelines for advanced life support (Box 11.1).

Box 11.1   Advanced cardiac life support guidelines

- No response, breathing or pulse—start CPR
- Call for help
- Ventilation: cardiac massage ratio of 1:5
- Precordial thump
- Place defibrillator paddles correctly
- Oxygenate
- Intubate
- Venous access

Further management when life support is established includes the following:

(1) If *no* intravenous access: adrenaline or atropine in double or triple doses down tracheal tube.
(2) In prolonged resuscitation, consider 50 mmol sodium bicarbonate (50 ml of 8·4% solution) according to arterial gas analysis.
(3) In post-resuscitation care:
    - monitor in intensive care or coronary care unit
    - check arterial gases, plasma electrolytes and chest X-ray.

There are three major types of arrhythmia: EMD (electromechanical dissociation—'QRS' without palpable pulse), ventricular fibrillation (or pulseless ventricular tachycardia), and asystole. The management of these three irregularities is described below.

Electromechanical dissociation

(1) Consider following causes and treat appropriately:
  - hypovolaemia
  - tension pneumothorax
  - cardiac tamponade
  - pulmonary embolism
  - drug overdosage
  - hypothermia
  - electrolyte imbalance.
(2) Adrenaline 1 mg intravenously.
(3) 10 CPR sequences of 5:1 compression/ventilation.
(4) *Loop* of steps 2 and 3 above.
(5) Consider:
  - pressor agents
  - calcium
  - alkalinising agents
  - adrenaline 5 mg intravenously.

Ventricular fibrillation

(1) Precordial thump.
(2) DC shock 200 joules (J).
(3) DC shock 200 J.
(4) DC shock 360 J.
(5) Adrenaline 1 mg intravenously.
(6) 10 CPR sequences of 5:1 compression/ventilation.
(7) DC shock 360 J.
(8) DC shock 360 J.
(9) DC shock 360 J.
(10) *Loop* of steps 5 to 9 above.
(11) Time between the 3rd and 4th DC shock should not be >2 minutes.
(12) Adrenaline should be given every 2–3 min.
(13) Continue *loops* for as long as defibrillation indicated.
(14) After *3 loops* consider:
  - alkalinising agents
  - antiarrhythmic drugs.

Asystole

(1) Precordial thump.
(2a) *If* ventricular fibrillation NOT excluded:
  - DC shock 200 J

- DC shock 200 J
- DC shock 360 J.

(2b) *If* ventricular fibrillation excluded:
   - adrenaline 1 mg intravenously
   - 10 CPR sequences of 5:1 compression/ventilation
   - atropine 3 mg intravenously ONCE only.

(3) Electrical activity evident:
   - no—return to step 2(b)
   - yes—pace.

(4) If no response after 3 cycles:
   - consider adrenaline 5 mg.

A surgeon may be able to do internal cardiac massage if the chest or the abdomen is already opened, but this will depend on their expertise.

Transfer to the intensive care unit should only be made when the patient is stable and with full monitoring devices attached.

Paediatric resuscitation

You should start cardiopulmonary resuscitation in infants (<1 year old) if the brachial pulse is less than 60 beats/min. Two fingers are placed on the lower sternum and compressions undertaken at a rate of 100 per minute to a depth of about 2 cm. Infants need an endotracheal tube size <4·0 mm diameter.

Children (>1 year) require the heel of one hand on the lower sternum with compressions at a rate of 100 per minute to a depth of 3 cm. The size of endotracheal tube for children is age (years)/4 + 4·5 mm.

Management steps for asystole are listed below.

(1) Ventilate with 100% O_2.
(2) Use intravenous or intraosseous access.
(3) Give adrenaline 10 µg/kg.
(4) Give CPR for 3 minutes.
(5) Give adrenaline 100 µg/kg.
(6) *Loop* steps 4 and 5.
(7) Consider i.v. fluids or alkalinising agents or both.
(8) Give adrenaline dose × 10, down endotracheal tube if no intravenous access.

Management steps for ventricular fibrillation are listed below.

(1) Give precordial thump.
(2) Defibrillate 2 J/kg.
(3) Defibrillate 2 J/kg.
(4) Defibrillate 4 J/kg.
(5) Ventilate with 100% O_2; establish intravenous or intraosseous access.

(6) Give adrenaline 10 µg/kg.

(7) Give CPR 1 min.

(8) Defibrillate 4 J/kg.

(9) Defibrillate 4 J/kg.

(10) Defibrillate 4 J/kg.

(11) Consider electrolytes, drugs, hypothermia.

(12) Give adrenaline 100 µg/kg.

(13) *Loop* steps 7 to 12.

(14) Give adrenaline dose × 10, down endotracheal tube if no other access.

(15) After 3 loops consider alkalinising agents or antiarrhythmic drugs, or both.

Management steps for electromechanical dissociation (EMD) are listed below. The same causes should be excluded as in adults (p. 53).

(1) Look for cause and treat appropriately.

(2) Ventilate with 100% oxygen.

(3) Use intravenous or intraosseous access.

(4) Give adrenaline 10 µg/kg.

(5) Give intravenous fluids 20 ml/kg.

(6) Give CPR 3 min.

(7) Give adrenaline 100 µg/kg.

(8) *Loop* steps 6 and 7.

(9) Give adrenaline dose × 10, down tracheal tube after 90 s if no i.v. access.

Adrenaline ampoules are available at concentrations of 1 in 1000 and 1 in 10 000. It is important that the amount of adrenaline present in 1 ml of each concentration is known, so that the correct doses can be given at a cardiac arrest.

$$1:1000 = 1 \text{ g in } 1000 \text{ ml}$$
$$= 1000 \text{ mg in } 1000 \text{ ml}$$
$$= 1 \text{ mg in } 1 \text{ ml}$$

$$1:10\,000 = 1 \text{ g in } 10\,000 \text{ ml}$$
$$= 1000 \text{ mg in } 10\,000 \text{ ml}$$
$$= 1 \text{ mg in } 10 \text{ ml}$$
$$= 1000 \text{ µg in } 10 \text{ ml}$$
$$= 100 \text{ µg in } 1 \text{ ml}$$

Therefore, there is 1 mg adrenaline in 1 ml of 1 in 1000 or 10 ml of 1 in 10 000.

Conclusion

The success rate of resuscitation in hospital, as assessed by the number of patients returning home, remains disappointing. The prompt recognition and management of the arrest is essential and, if it occurs during anaesthesia, the cause must be identified and treated.

The rapid establishment of ventilation of the lungs with oxygen and vascular access is essential for successful resuscitation. Your anaesthetic skills often make you the natural leader of the arrest team.

12: Haemorrhage and blood transfusion

Estimation of blood loss

Surgeons cause blood loss and it is in their nature always to underestimate that loss. As an anaesthetist you must try to assess accurately the amount of blood shed and replace it with an appropriate intravenous solution. There are four main ways of estimating blood loss (Box 12.1).

> ### Box 12.1 Blood loss estimation
> - Clinical observation
> - Weighing of swabs
> - Volume of suction
> - Dilution techniques

During surgery it is a useful exercise to try to guess how much blood has been lost before checking with the estimate derived from weighing the swabs and measuring the volume of suction. With practice, your guess will become reasonably accurate for a known surgeon. However, this method should not be relied on and can be hopelessly inaccurate when you start working with a new surgical team.

Apart from surgical spillage, it is important to remember that, in trauma, patients will have occult loss in limb and pelvic fractures, and in chest or abdominal injuries.

Swab weighing relies on the principle that 1 ml of blood weighs approximately 1 g. A 3×4 in swab weighs 20 g when dry and about 35 g when saturated. This 15 g difference represents about 15 ml of blood. An 18×18 in swab contains about 150 ml of blood when saturated. Three of these large swabs full of blood contain about 450 ml, which is equivalent to 1 unit of blood.

The volume of fluid in the suction apparatus may contain surgical "washing fluid" as well as blood. This overestimate is a useful precaution as the amount of blood on the surgical drapes, down the surgeons and on the floor cannot be measured. In major surgery it can easily be equivalent to 1–2 units of blood.

Dilution techniques are rarely used in clinical practice but rely on the measurement of the concentration of haemoglobin in the suction fluid to calculate the blood loss.

Patients should be transfused according to cardiovascular variables rather than relying on the estimates of blood loss. The heart rate, arterial pressure and central venous pressure are obvious guides and the measurement of the haematocrit or haemoglobin may be useful. A haemoglobin concentration of 10 g/dl, or a haematocrit of 30%, is often considered the lower limit of adequate oxygen delivery, even when the circulating blood volume and cardiac output are maintained. Although this limit is arbitrary, we have found it a useful practical guide and will transfuse red cells unless there are obvious contraindications. Lower values of 25% haematocrit or 8 g/dl haemoglobin concentration have been proposed, but there is then little physiological reserve if further rapid blood loss occurs.

Blood and blood products

Storage

Blood after donation is immediately cooled to 4–6°C. These temperature limits must be rigidly observed to preserve the red cells and minimise the multiplication of chance bacterial contaminants. Blood from the refrigerator should be used within 30 minutes.

A unit (500 ml) of blood is collected into a bag which contains 70 ml of citrate, phosphate, and dextrose (CPD) solution. The plasma is commonly centrifuged off for other use. The red cells are then suspended in a saline, adenine, glucose and mannitol (SAG-M) solution. The purpose of the storage additives is shown in Box 12.2.

Box 12.2   Additives used in red cell storage

- Citrate: chelates calcium
- Phosphate: maintains ATP, reduces haemolysis and increases red cell survival
- Saline: decreases viscosity of red cell concentrates
- Adenine: maintains ATP, improves red cell mobility
- Glucose: energy for red cells, decreases hydrolysis of ATP
- Mannitol: reduces haemolysis

Whole blood is devoid of functioning platelets after 2–3 days of storage and the clotting factors V and VIII are reduced to 10% of normal within 24 hours. Although adequate amounts of the coagulation factors I, II, VII,

IX, X, XI, XII are present in whole blood, red cell concentrates contain virtually no coagulation factors.

Potassium concentrations rise progressively in stored blood and can reach up to 30 mmol/l after 3 weeks. Following transfusion, viable red cells re-establish their ionic pumping mechanism and intracellular uptake of potassium occurs rapidly. Blood $\geqslant 3$ weeks old is acidic with pH values down to 6·6 and this results mainly from the lactic acid generated by red cell metabolism.

Preparations

There are about twenty different types of blood and blood products available for adult and paediatric use. The main ones used by anaesthetists are shown in Box 12.3.

Box 12.3 Blood products in common use

Blood/blood product	Volume (ml) per unit	Storage temperature (°C)	Shelf life
• Whole blood	500	4–6	35 days
• Red cell concentrates	300	4–6	35 days
• Fresh frozen plasma	150	−30	1 year
• Platelet concentrates	50	22	5 days
• Cryoprecipitate	18	−30	1 year

Fresh frozen plasma (FFP) contains all the components of the coagulation, fibrinolytic, and complement systems. In addition it also has proteins that maintain oncotic pressure, fats, and carbohydrates.

Cryoprecipitate contains factor VIII and fibrinogen.

Complications of blood transfusion

Complications of blood transfusion include those listed in Box 12.4.

Physical

Circulatory overload should be avoided by the judicious transfusion of blood according to the measured cardiovascular variables such as arterial pressure, central venous pressure, and heart rate. Air embolism can occur from errors in blood administration, particularly when the bags are pressurised. Microaggregates are platelet and white cell debris which are

---

Box 12.4 Blood transfusion complications

- Physical
  - circulatory overload
  - embolism (air, microaggregates)
  - hypothermia

- Immunological
  - pyrogenic
  - type I hypersensitivity
  - graft versus host reactions

- Biochemical
  - acid base disturbances
  - hyperkalaemia
  - citrate toxicity
  - impaired oxygen release

- Infective

- Haemolytic transfusion reactions

- Disseminated intravascular coagulation

---

removed by the use of 20–40 μm blood filters. These filters are either screen or depth in nature. Reduced transfusion of microaggregates may result in a decreased incidence of nonhaemolytic, febrile reactions, and less pulmonary injury and histamine release. Depth filters cause impaction and absorption of microaggregates and screen filters operate by direct interception of the microemboli. Blood filters cause increased resistance to blood flow, haemolysis, complement activation, and can deplete the blood of any remaining viable platelets. We do not believe that their value has been proven and never use them.

Anaesthetised patients have impaired temperature regulation and the rapid transfusion of cold blood exacerbates the hypothermia. The value of warming blood during transfusion has been demonstrated repeatedly and should be undertaken on every occasion.

Immunological

Pyrogenic reactions can occur in the recipient to white cell antigens or the polysaccharide products of bacterial metabolism. Rarely gram negative bacteria exist in stored blood. Plasma proteins are responsible for any anaphylactic or allergic reactions that happen. These reactions are rare, and range from severe hypotension to mild rashes. "Graft versus host" reactions are caused by blood containing HLA-incompatible, immunocompetent lymphocytes given to patients with immunosuppression.

Pyrexia may develop and the disease can be fatal without suitable transfusion precautions.

It has been suggested, but is unproven, that patients with malignancy requiring transfusion have a greater risk of a recurrence.

Biochemical

The rapid infusion of large volumes of stored blood may result in acidosis in the recipient. This is particularly likely to occur if the liver is unable to metabolise the lactate and citrate because of inadequate hepatic perfusion, hypothermia, and even hepatic disease. A persistent acidosis decreases myocardial function. A temporary improvement in cardiac output often follows the use of intravenous calcium chloride in these circumstances, although there is no obvious relationship to plasma ionised calcium values. The restoration of normal liver function usually corrects the problem.

Depletion of 2,3-diphosphoglycerate (DPG) in the red cells shifts the oxygen dissociation curve to the left and oxygen is released less easily from transfused blood. Modern additives have improved the concentration of 2,3-DPG for up to 14 days, and 25% of cells are back to normal function in 3 hours and 50% in 24 hours.

Infective

All blood products except albumin and gamma globulin can transmit infectious diseases. Hepatitis B, C, syphilis, and HIV are screened for, but cytomegalovirus, malaria, Epstein–Barr virus, and parvovirus infection can be transmitted following transfusion.

Haemolytic transfusion reactions

Acute, haemolytic, pyrogenic reactions usually occur due to *errors* in the clerical administration of blood. However, blood group and rhesus incompatibility can also result in severe haemolytic reactions. Blood should be checked by two people against the patient's identity band. The recipient's name, hospital number, blood group, and blood expiry date must be checked and signed for. In practice, during emergency work, it is often not possible for two people to check the blood and it is then *imperative that you slowly and deliberately check each unit.* Sometimes you have the opportunity to check all the blood before inducing anaesthesia.

Disseminated intravascular coagulation (DIC)

DIC is widespread activation of the coagulation and fibrinolytic systems which results in clotting throughout the whole vasculature. It has many possible causes, but can occur in 30% of cases of massive transfusion. It presents primarily as a haemorrhagic disorder caused by loss of platelets and soluble clotting factors (especially fibrinogen).

61

Massive blood transfusion

Various definitions exist for this term. It is normally defined in one of three ways:

- acute administration of >1·5 times the estimated blood volume;
- the replacement of the patient's total blood volume by stored bank blood in <24 hours;
- the acute administration of more than 10% of the blood volume in <10 minutes.

Formulae for estimating the blood volume are shown in Box 12.5.

Box 12.5   Blood volume formulae

- Neonate 90 ml/kg
- Infants 2 years of age 80 ml/kg
- Adult male 70 ml/kg
- Adult female 60 ml/kg

It is recommended that, after a 6-unit transfusion, a set of basic screening tests is undertaken to exclude DIC. These are:

- haemoglobin and platelet count;
- prothrombin time (PT) and activated partial thromboplastin time (APTT);
- plasma fibrinogen concentration;
- fibrin degradation products;
- pH from arterial blood gas analysis.

The diagnosis of DIC is made by noting the trend:

- increase: APTT, PT, fibrin degradation products;
- decrease: platelet count, fibrinogen concentration.

The correction of these abnormalities is made after haematological consultation.

The abnormalities in PT and APTT are normally corrected by the administration of FFP (4 units). A low platelet count should be restored to above $100 \times 10^9/l$ by the administration of 6–8 packs of platelets. Low fibrinogen levels are treated with cryoprecipitate aiming for a level of >1 g/l (normal 2–4·5 g/l). If the patient has an arterial pH <7·2 and is continuing to bleed, the administration of 50 mmol bicarbonate (50 ml of 8·4% solution) should be considered.

Conclusion

Surgery results in blood loss. You must know how to estimate this loss, understand the blood products available and be able to use cardiovascular and haematological monitoring to transfuse them appropriately. Think of blood as another potent drug that you will give frequently. It must be checked carefully before use, it can be life-saving, but also has unwanted side effects.

13: Anaphylactic reactions

Whilst minor allergic reactions are not uncommon in anaesthesia, major anaphylactic reactions are rare. Prompt treatment, with the emphasis on the early use of adrenaline will usually lead to a successful outcome.

An anaphylactic reaction is an exaggerated response to a foreign protein or substance to which previous exposure and sensitisation has occurred. Histamine, serotonin and other vasoactive substances are liberated in response to an IgE-mediated reaction.

An anaphylactoid reaction results in the same clinical manifestations as an anaphylactic reaction, but is not mediated by a sensitising IgE antibody. Previous exposure to a drug will not have occurred, but susceptible individuals often have a history of allergies.

Every anaesthetist should know and practise an "anaphylaxis drill". The clinical manifestations of severe allergic reactions are shown in Box 13.1.

Although all anaesthetic drugs can cause severe allergic reactions, the neuromuscular blocking drugs account for the majority of the triggering agents. Only about a third of these patients will have had previous exposure to the specific drug. Latex hypersensitivity is an increasing

---

Box 13.1 Signs of severe allergic drug reactions

- Pruritis
- Flushing
- Erythema
- Nausea, vomiting, and diarrhoea
- Angioedema
- Laryngeal oedema with stridor
- Bronchospasm with wheeze
- Hypotension
- Cardiovascular collapse
- Disseminated intravascular coagulation
- Sudden death

cause of anaphylaxis and is found commonly 30–60 min after the start of surgery.

Females are more likely to have a reaction than males.

Treatment

The management of an anaphylactic reaction should be considered in two stages:

- immediate treatment;
- secondary treatment.

The following guidelines assume that the patient is a 70 kg adult in whom the diagnosis is not in doubt.

Immediate management (Box 13.2).

Box 13.2   Anaphylaxis—immediate management

- Stop administration of suspected drug, if possible.
- Call for HELP.
- Stop anaesthesia and surgery if feasible.
- Maintain airway.
- Give *100% oxygen* (consider intubation and ventilation).
- Give intravenous *adrenaline* (especially if bronchospasm present):
  - 0·5–1·0 ml of 1:10 000 (50–100 μg) aliquots
  - 5–8 μg/min if prolonged therapy required.
- Start intravascular volume replacement by colloid 10 ml/kg.
- Consider cardiopulmonary resuscitation.

A reduction in peripheral vascular resistance and a loss of intravascular volume are the initial pathophysiological changes. Fluid therapy is important for resuscitation and central venous pressure measurement may be necessary; however the priority is intravenous adrenaline.

Secondary management (Box 13.3).

It is important to remember in the secondary management of these patients that intensive care facilities may be needed, and that in prolonged treatment awareness can occur and should be prevented.

Box 13.3   Anaphylaxis—secondary management

- Adrenaline-resistant bronchospasm. Consider:
  - intravenous salbutamol 250 μg loading dose and 5–20 μg/min maintenance, *or*
  - aminophylline 4–8 mg/kg over 20 min.

- Bronchospasm and/or cardiovascular collapse. Consider:
  - intravenous hydrocortisone 300 mg, *or*
  - methyl prednisolone 2 g.

- Antihistamines. Consider:
  - intravenous chlorpheniramine 20 mg diluted, administer slowly.

- After 20 minutes and severe acidosis present. Consider:
  - sodium bicarbonate.

- Catecholamine infusions. Consider:
  - adrenaline 5 mg in 500 ml (10 μg/ml) at rate 10–85 ml/h, *or*
  - noradrenaline 4 mg in 500 ml (8 μg/ml) at rate 25–100 ml/h.

- Consider coagulopathy: clotting screen.

- Arterial gas analysis for oxygenation and degree of acidosis.

Investigations

After a severe allergic drug reaction, the patient must be investigated thoroughly and both the patient and the general practitioner informed of the results. This is usually carried out in consultation with a clinical immunologist. The investigations normally take place in the order below.

(1) Blood tests for confirmation of allergic reaction.
(2) Full anaesthetic history.
(3) Skin tests.
(4) Patient reporting: hazard card, Medic-alert bracelet.
(5) Report to Committee on Safety of Medicines.

At the time of the reaction, serial blood samples are taken for serum tryptase (a neutral protease released from mast cells), complement activation, and IgE antibody concentrations. These will confirm that a reaction has occurred, but will not identify the causative agent.

After a full medical history and a delay of at least four weeks, a "skin prick test" is undertaken. This correctly identifies most causative agents. Full resuscitation equipment must be available and detailed protocols have been described, indicating appropriate dilutions of drugs and the use of control solutions.

The case must be reported to the Committee on Safety of Medicines. The patient should carry a written record of the reaction and either an anaesthetic hazard card or a Medic-alert bracelet.

Conclusion

Life-threatening anaphylaxis is a rare complication of anaesthesia. A knowledge of the immediate and secondary management must be learnt during the early months of training. The mainstay of immediate treatment is intravenous adrenaline. Remember:

ANAPHYLAXIS = ADRENALINE

14: Malignant hyperthermia

Malignant hyperthermia (MH) is a rare complication of general anaesthesia which results from an abnormal increase in muscle metabolism in response to all potent inhalational agents and suxamethonium. There is often a family history of death or major problems associated with anaesthesia, and the gene is inherited as an autosomal dominant. Even with the ready availability of a specific therapeutic drug, dantrolene, deaths from MH still occur, mostly because of a failure to recognise the onset of the syndrome. If you are lucky, you will never see a patient with MH, but we know an anaesthetist who induced MH in three patients within five years! The main reason why this rare syndrome provokes so much attention is because, like anaphylaxis, it is one of those occasions when an anaesthetic drug can kill the patient.

The primary defect in MH is in the sarcoplasmic reticulum of skeletal muscle. Abnormal increases in calcium ion concentration occur on exposure to triggering agents and this biochemical change results in acidosis, heat production, and muscle stiffness.

Estimates of the incidence of MH vary, but a figure of 1:10 000 to 1:50 000 is commonly cited. This value represents typical practice in a district general hospital, but there is an increased incidence in the following groups:

- males
- children and young adults
- patients with congenital musculoskeletal disorders.

Thus, if you work in a major orthopaedic centre which undertakes scoliosis surgery in adolescents, you are more likely to encounter the problem.

It is helpful to try to identify MH before surgery by noting the following points:

- family history of problems or sudden death associated with general anaesthesia;
- increased circulating creatine kinase (CK) concentration;
- *in vitro* testing of muscle biopsy to caffeine and halothane.

Unfortunately, circulating CK concentrations are of limited use. They may be normal in MH-susceptible patients and there are many other causes of an increased CK concentration. Nevertheless, if there is a family history of MH and the patient has an abnormally raised CK without obvious cause, they are likely to be MH-susceptible. *In vitro* testing of a muscle biopsy is, at present, the most accurate method of diagnosing MH and is undertaken only in specialised centres. The patient is described as MHS (susceptible), MHN (normal), or MHE (equivocal). MHE means that they respond positively to either halothane or caffeine, but not both.

MH is triggered by all volatile anaesthetic drugs and suxamethonium. The response to the administration of suxamethonium at induction of anaesthesia is abnormal in some MH-susceptible patients. Instead of the usual fasciculations followed by muscle relaxation, there are vigorous fasciculations with failure to relax and, in particular, masseter spasm. This spasm makes opening the mouth difficult and so endotracheal intubation may be a problem. The occurrence of masseter spasm should be treated as an important prognostic indicator of possible MH susceptibility (approximately 50%). Management is undertaken as shown below:

(1) HELP.
(2) Halt anaesthesia.
(3) *Do not give volatile agents.*
(4) Elective surgery: abandon and monitor patient.
(5) Emergency surgery:
   - follow advice
   - monitor patient
   - use "safe" techniques (box 14.4)
   - prepare to treat MH
   - perform arterial gas analysis early and regularly.

The key feature is *not to administer potent volatile agents.* Suxamethonium alone usually results in a relatively mild, self-limiting MH, whereas the combination of suxamethonium with a volatile anaesthetic is a potent trigger.

Presentation

There are no obvious signs of the onset of MH, other than an abnormal response to suxamethonium. The main clinical signs are shown in Box 14.1.

Box 14.1 Clinical signs of MH

- Abnormal response to suxamethonium (masseter spasm)
- Tachycardia (possibly arrhythmias)
- Tachypnoea
- Increased use of soda-lime
- Peripheral cyanosis
- Muscle stiffness
- Patient feels hot

The peripheral circulation is often decreased in MH due to the marked increase in catecholamine secretion, so do not wait for the brow to feel hot—it may never happen! The metabolic signs of MH are more obvious and reflect the massive stimulation of muscle metabolism (Box 14.2).

Box 14.2   Metabolic signs of MH

- Acidosis
  - increased CO_2 production
  - increased lactic acid production
- Hyperkalaemia
- Haemoconcentration
- Hyperglycaemia
- Hypoxaemia
- Hyperthermia

The earliest objective sign of the onset of MH is increased CO_2 production as shown by a raised end-tidal CO_2 concentration with capnography. Body temperature is not a reliable sign, unless a good estimate of core temperature is available (not rectal). The metabolic changes provide the basis for the confirmation of the suspected diagnosis. Arterial gas analysis should be undertaken and in established MH will show a severe acidosis, both respiratory and metabolic, and often hyperkalaemia. Once the diagnosis of MH has been confirmed, then correct treatment must be started immediately.

Treatment

The treatment of MH can be considered as specific therapy with dantrolene and general supportive management (Box 14.3).

Box 14.3   Overall management plan for MH

- Specific treatment
  - dantrolene

- General supportive therapy
  - acidosis
  - hyperkalaemia
  - haemoconcentration
  - arrhythmias
  - hyperthermia

Dantrolene must be administered promptly and the following guidelines have been found to be effective.

(1) Discontinue volatile agents and terminate surgery, if possible.
(2) Hyperventilate with 100% O_2 (2–3 times minute volume). Use opioid + benzodiazepine to maintain unconsciousness.
(3) Correct metabolic acidosis (at least 100 mmol bicarbonate).
(4) Dantrolene 1 mg/kg i.v. every 10 min until MH controlled. Assess therapy by:
  ● arterial gas analysis
  ● tachycardia
  ● muscle stiffness
  ● temperature.
(5) Establish appropriate monitoring.
(6) Correct hyperkalaemia and rehydrate.
(7) Treat severe tachycardia (small dose of beta-blocking drug).
(8) Cool if necessary (infants and children only).
(9) Induce diuresis when rehydrated.
(10) Monitor carefully for 24 hours (ITU).

Dantrolene is difficult to dissolve and it can take a long time to form a solution. Once it is in suspension, use it. Fortunately dantrolene works rapidly and 1 mg/kg is often sufficient to stop the hypermetabolism within a few minutes. Most patients require a total dose of only 1–2 mg/kg.

Do not waste time on cooling the patient unless it is an infant or child; thermogenesis will cease once the MH is controlled.

Anaesthesia for MH-susceptible patients

It is much easier to manage MH if you are aware of the problem before the anaesthetic. A "safe" technique means avoiding the potent volatile agents and suxamethonium and using a "clean" anaesthetic machine. This is obtained by removing the vaporisers, changing all disposable tubing and then purging the machine with 10 l of O_2 for 10 min. Regional or general anaesthesia may be used (Box 14.4).

Full monitoring must be undertaken—capnography, oxygen consumption, temperature measurement and often the intravascular measurement of arterial pressure and central venous pressure.

Conclusion

Malignant hyperthermia is not easy to diagnose. Although it is rare, the possibility of MH must be considered if you find an unexpected increase

---

Box 14.4   Anaesthesia in suspected MH

- Regional anaesthesia
  - all drugs safe
- General anaesthesia
  - premedication: benzodiazepine, opiates
  - induction: all i.v. drugs safe
  - neuromuscular blockade: all non-depolarising drugs safe
  - maintenance: N_2O–O_2—total intravenous

---

in CO_2 excretion, tachycardia, or tachypnoea during anaesthesia. The diagnosis is confirmed by arterial gas analysis. Dantrolene is effective if given early: know where it is kept in theatre—one day you may need it urgently.

15: Stridor—upper airway obstruction

Acute stridor is a life-threatening emergency. It usually occurs in children, but is occasionally found in adults. Complete obstruction of the upper airway may occur rapidly and the change from partial to complete obstruction is often unpredictable. Upper airway obstruction will lead to fatigue and respiratory failure if left untreated and pulmonary oedema may result from prolonged airway obstruction.

The common causes of airway obstruction are shown (Box 15.1).

Box 15.1   Common causes of upper airway obstruction

- Congenital
- Acquired
  - infective
    - laryngotracheobronchitis (croup)
    - epiglottitis
  - traumatic
    - burns/smoke inhalation
    - foreign body inhalation
    - postintubation laryngospasm/oedema
  - neoplastic

Laryngospasm and postintubation oedema are considered in Chapter 17.

Clinical presentation

Inspiratory stridor occurs when the obstruction is at or above the level of the cricoid ring. Expiratory stridor, wheeze and chest hyperinflation are found with lower intrathoracic obstruction (for example, foreign body).

Stridor is seen initially on exertion but, as the obstruction worsens, it occurs at rest. Children often prefer to sit and there is hyperextension of the neck in an effort to prevent airway collapse. Chest recession and the use of the accessory muscles of respiration occurs. Drooling results from a failure to swallow saliva. There is a gradual loss of interest in the surroundings and a reduced level of consciousness (Box 15.2).

Box 15.2 Symptoms and signs of upper airway obstruction

- Type of stridor: inspiratory/expiratory
- Barking cough
- Hoarseness
- Chest recession
- Accessory muscle usage
- Sitting forwards position
- Nasal flaring
- Hyperextension of neck
- Drooling
- Tachycardia
- Tachypnoea
- Cyanosis
- Loss of interest
- Reduced consciousness

Box 15.3 Syracuse croup assessment scoring system

Symptoms and signs	Score			
	0	1	2	3
Stridor	none	faintly audible	easily audible	—
Cyanosis	none	minimal	obvious	—
Sternal retraction	none	present	—	—
Respiratory rate/min				
0–5 kg	<35	36–40	41–45	>45
5–10 kg	<30	31–35	36–40	>40
>10 kg	<20	21–24	25–30	>30
Heart rate/min				
<3 months	<150	151–165	166–190	>190
3–6 months	<130	131–145	146–170	>170
7–12 months	<120	121–135	136–150	>150
1–3 years	<110	111–125	126–140	>140
3–5 years	<90	91–100	101–120	>120

A score >5 indicates intensive care admission.
A score ≤5 is considered safe for transfer to a paediatric ward.

Diagnosis

Scoring systems have been devised for specific causes of airway obstruction such as croup and give some indication of the severity of the disease (Box 15.3). They may, however, lead to a false sense of security. Cyanosis is often difficult to detect and is an indication for urgent transfer to an intensive care unit.

A concise and relevant history with repeated, frequent examinations of the child should be made. A past history of *Haemophilus influenza* type b (Hib) vaccination makes epiglottitis an unlikely, but not impossible, diagnosis. Quiet observation of the child from a distance will often provide all the necessary information. A chest X-ray is rarely necessary and *should only be done in the intensive care unit*, as appropriate resuscitation facilities must be available. This usually precludes the radiology department at night.

Pulse oximetry (>94% saturation on air) may confirm adequate oxygenation but arterial gas analysis is unhelpful. It will certainly upset the child, exacerbate the condition, and may delay treatment. If you have any doubts about the severity of the obstruction, admit the child to the intensive care unit and accompany the child yourself.

Laryngotracheobronchitis (croup)

Croup affects the whole respiratory tract, but oedema of the glottic and subglottic region causes the airway obstruction. The aetiology is:

- viral-parainfluenza, respiratory syncytial, mycoplasmic pneumonia;
- bacterial;
- spasmodic.

The child (mean age about 18 months) usually has a history of an upper respiratory tract infection with moderate fever for 48 hours before the onset of stridor. Stridor is often worse at night and stridor at rest is an indication for hospital admission.

The principles of care are:

(1) Give adequate hydration.
(2) Give paracetamol elixir 15 mg/kg 6-hourly.
(3) Give nebulised adrenaline 0·5 ml/kg 1:1000 (maximum 5 ml) every 1–4 hours depending on severity. Monitor with ECG.
(4) Worsening respiratory distress, reduced consciousness, and failure to respond to adrenaline is indication for endotracheal intubation.
(5) Steroids decrease the duration of intubation.

Bacterial tracheitis, commonly from *Staphylococcus aureus*, requires antibiotic treatment (for example, cefotaxime 50 mg/kg every 6 hours). Spasmodic croup occurs suddenly at night without a pre-existing infection. There is a dramatic response to nebulised adrenaline, and dexamethasone 0·6 mg/kg is also effective.

75

Epiglottitis

This is caused mainly by *Haemophilus influenza* type b infection and classically occurs in the 2–7-year-old group. The incidence has declined dramatically since vaccination programmes have been implemented. The history is typically short. There is a high fever, malaise, dysphagia, dysphonia, an absent cough, and the stridor has a unique, low-pitched, snoring quality. The child will sit with an open mouth. Antibiotic therapy should be started and, if there is a high risk of obstruction, an artificial airway should be inserted. If complete obstruction occurs before intubation, hand ventilation is usually possible despite the oedematous structures.

Foreign body

Some foreign bodies will pass down into the bronchi, usually the right, but others will lodge in the larynx causing obstruction and the risk of an hypoxic arrest. The European Resuscitation Council recommends the following treatment:

- Infants <1 year: five back blows between shoulder blades with the head lower than the trunk and the child prone; if this does not work, five chest thrusts with the child supine can be given.
- Children >1 year: if the above is unsuccessful, then abdominal thrusts with the child supine (Heimlich manoeuvre) can be performed.

In a life-threatening situation, a foreign body in the laryngeal area can be removed under direct vision using a laryngoscope and a pair of Magill intubating forceps. It should only be attempted by an experienced anaesthetist.

Management of intubation

If a child is deteriorating, or unresponsive to treatment, endotracheal intubation to bypass the obstruction must be undertaken. The principles of management are shown below:

(1) Get HELP: an *experienced anaesthetist* is needed.
(2) ENT surgeon should be present if possible. ?tracheostomy.
(3) Transfer the child to theatre/intensive care unit.
(4) Supervise transfer and take resuscitation equipment.
(5) Keep parents present and informed.
(6) Induce anaesthesia via inhalational route, oxygen, and halothane.
(7) Insert intravenous cannula *after* induction.
(8) Give atropine 20 μg/kg i.v..
(9) Monitor fully.
(10) Use full range of endotracheal tubes—smaller than expected for age.
(11) Secure tracheal tube. ?Change to nasal.
(12) Transfer from theatre to intensive care unit if necessary.

(13) ?Sedate child.
(14) Humidify inspired gases.
(15) Maintain good airway toilet.

It is important not to upset the child as this may precipitate complete obstruction of the airway, and for this reason intravenous cannulation should not be attempted until after induction of anaesthesia.

A principle of anaesthesia that is *absolute* is that neuromuscular blocking drugs must *not* be used if there are any doubts about the patency of the upper airway (ability to ventilate the lungs) or the ease of intubation. A patient who is impossible to ventilate and intubate will die of hypoxia if they are paralysed. In this situation endotracheal intubation must be undertaken using either local anaesthetic techniques or inhalational anaesthesia. If an inhalational technique is used, it is imperative that intubation is not attempted until deep anaesthesia has been achieved. Alternatively the airway may be secured by a tracheostomy or cricothyroid puncture. In children with upper airway obstruction, inhalational anaesthesia is the chosen method and this may take up to 15 minutes.

Atropine is given to block the bradycardia that may occur during intubation. The tracheal tube must not be allowed to come out as this causes much excitement amongst the staff. It should be well secured to prevent an alert child from pulling it out unexpectedly—children are often sedated.

The tracheal tube can be removed when the child has recovered from the infection and there is a leak around the tube indicating that the oedema has subsided.

Conclusion

Stridor is a medical emergency that needs assistance from an experienced anaesthetist. A trainee must know the principles of treatment of maintaining a patent airway in this situation. If you have any doubts about the severity of the obstruction, transfer the child to an intensive care unit and accompany them on transfer. Stay calm—you are dealing with a frightened child, very worried parents and a paediatrician who often knows less about an obstructed airway than you.

16: Pneumothorax

A pneumothorax is defined as the presence of air within the pleural cavity. For it to occur, a communication between the pleural cavity, and either the tracheobronchial tree or the atmosphere by a defect in the chest wall must be present. The main causes are shown in Box 16.1.

Box 16.1   Causes of pneumothorax

- Spontaneous: asthma, Marfan's syndrome
- Iatrogenic: central venous catheters, surgery (for example, nephrectomy)
- Traumatic: fractured ribs, other thoracic trauma

An emergency arises when a *tension pneumothorax* develops. This is most likely to occur when intermittent positive pressure ventilation is applied to the lungs of patients with the following problems:

- undiagnosed spontaneous pneumothorax;
- emphysema;
- lung bullae;
- asthma.

It is important to remember that all patients have the potential to develop a pneumothorax in anaesthesia. The situation is exacerbated by the fact that nitrous oxide diffuses rapidly into gas-filled spaces and thus increases the size of any pneumothorax.

In a tension pneumothorax air entering the pleural cavity is unable to return to the lung and increases the pressure in the hemithorax causing lung collapse. The mediastinum is shifted across the midline, decreasing venous return and impeding cardiac output, with impaired ventilation to the other lung. This combination of major physiological changes is potentially lethal.

The diagnosis is not easy, but should be suspected when the signs shown in Box 16.2 occur during or shortly after anaesthesia.

Treatment

If time allows, a chest X-ray in expiration will confirm the diagnosis. Nitrous oxide should be discontinued. A chest drain must be inserted. In a life-threatening situation a 14-gauge cannula should be inserted into the

> **Box 16.2   Signs of pneumothorax in anaesthesia**
>
> - Unexplained cyanosis
> - Wheeze
> - "Silent" chest on auscultation
> - Difficulty with ventilation
> - High airway pressures
> - Sudden change in airway pressures
> - Tachycardia
> - Hypotension

pleural cavity to relieve the tension pneumothorax. This must then be connected to an underwater drainage system.

A chest drainage tube is inserted into the second intercostal space in the midclavicular line or the fifth intercostal space in the midaxillary line. It is important to insert the tube through a *high* intercostal space. One author managed to place a right-sided chest drain using the transhepatic route, which was associated with a spectacular blood loss. Prompt surgery saved the patient. The important features of inserting a chest drain are stated below.

(1) Use an aseptic technique.
(2) If patient is unanaesthetised, inject local anaesthetic from skin to periosteum.
(3) Make 2–3 cm horizontal incision.
(4) Make blunt dissection through the tissues until it is just over the top of the rib.
(5) Puncture the parietal pleural with the tip of a clamp and put a gloved finger into the incision to avoid injury to any organs and to clear the area of any adhesions or clots.
(6) Clamp end of tube and advance it through the pleura to the desired length.
(7) Connect tube to chest drain—the underwater tube should be placed <5 cm into the water to minimise resistance.
(8) Suture the tube in place and confirm position by a chest X-ray.

Conclusion

Pneumothorax is uncommon in anaesthesia but must be considered when certain signs arise unexpectedly during or after anaesthesia. It is particularly likely in operations in the renal area. A tension pneumothorax must be treated by the insertion of a chest drain or, if this is unavailable, a 14-gauge intravenous cannula may be used temporarily.

17: Common intraoperative problems

Problems occurring during anaesthesia and surgery must be considered in an appropriate way. For example, the onset of an arrhythmia during surgery may have an anaesthetic cause, or result from surgical stimulation. A disturbance of cardiac rhythm is not necessarily indicative of myocardial disease. If the arrhythmia is accompanied by sweating and hypertension it probably results from excessive sympathoadrenal activity. You must learn to consider the causation of intraoperative problems in the following order:

- anaesthetic
- surgical
- medical.

In particular, we recommend that the following safety check is undertaken whenever an unexpected problem arises:

- Is the anaesthetic machine working correctly?
- Are the gas flows correct?
- Is the circuit assembled correctly and working?
- Is the airway patent?

This fundamental principle of an anaesthetic cause, before a surgical cause, before a medical cause, cannot be overemphasised. The simple mechanistic approach that a bradycardia needs intravenous atropine will be fatal if the slow heart rate is a response to hypoxaemia following a disconnection within the circuit. Identifying the site of the disconnection and oxygenating the patient is the obvious priority. Common causes of intraoperative problems are shown in Box 17.1.

Some problems remain after anaesthetic and surgical causes have been eliminated and need specific treatment.

80

Box 17.1   Common causes of intraoperative problems

- Anaesthesia
  - exclude HYPOXIA
  - exclude HYPERCAPNIA
  - response to laryngoscopy and intubation?
  - correct rotameter settings?
  - correct use of volatile agents?
  - pain?
  - awareness?
  - drugs—correct? interactions?
  - adequate monitoring?
  - malignant hyperthermia?

- Surgery
  - reflex responses—eye, dental surgery, vagal stimulation?
  - retractors correctly sited?
  - haemorrhage—occult?

- Medical
  - specific diseases—cardiac?
  - undiagnosed disease—phaeochromocytoma?
  - electrolyte imbalance?
  - acid/base balance?

Arrhythmias

Ectopic beats

These are common during surgery and, if they are occasional with no effect on arterial pressure, can usually be ignored. Otherwise treatment is undertaken as shown in Box 17.2.

Box 17.2   Treatment of ectopic beats

- Atrial
  - no specific treatment

- Nodal
  - consider atropine in 0·3 mg increments to a maximum 3 mg

- Ventricular
  - consider lignocaine 50–100 mg i.v. as slow bolus followed by infusion of 10 mg/min for 20 minutes and then 1–2 mg/min

---

Bradycardias

Sinus bradycardia is common during anaesthesia, usually as the result of anaesthetic drugs or surgical stimulation. If these causes have been excluded, treatment is undertaken as shown in Box 17.3.

Box 17.3   Treatment of bradycardias

- Sinus
  - consider atropine 0·3 mg increments to a maximum 3 mg

- 1st degree heart block
  - consider atropine as above

- 2nd degree heart block
  - consider atropine as above
  - consider isoprenaline infusion (4 µg/ml)
  - consider pacing

- Complete heart block
  - cardiology opinion
  - consider isoprenaline infusion as above
  - consider pacing

Supraventricular tachycardias

These arrhythmias are often difficult to differentiate during anaesthesia and surgery and the commonest types are:

- atrial fibrillation;
- atrial flutter and atrial tachycardia;
- junctional tachycardia (nodal and atrioventricular).

Rapid atrial fibrillation develops occasionally during anaesthesia and, after exclusion of anaesthetic and surgical cases, is treated as shown in box 17.4.

Box 17.4   Treatment of new atrial fibrillation

(1) Consider amiodarone 300 mg as slow bolus followed by 600 mg in 1 hour.

(2) Consider digoxin 250–500 µg slowly.

(3) If severe hypotension, give synchronised DC cardioversion:
- 100 J
- 200 J
- 360 J.

Slow atrial fibrillation is managed by intravenous atropine or pacing.

Other supraventricular tachycardias are shown in box 17.5.

Box 17.5   Treatment of supraventricular tachycardias

(1) Perform vagal manoeuvres.

(2) Give adenosine 3 mg bolus and repeat if necessary every 1–2 min using 6 mg, then 12 mg, then 12 mg boli.

(3) *If no hypotension*, but evidence of heart failure and heart rate <200 beats/ minute, then choose from:

- esmolol 40 mg over 1 minute and infusion 4 mg/min
- verapamil 5–10 mg
- amiodarone 300 mg bolus over 15 minutes and 600 mg infusion in 1 hour.

(4) *If hypotension*, heart failure and heart rate ≥200 beats/min consider

- synchronised cardioversion 100 J, then 200 J, then 360 J
- amiodarone 300 mg over 15 minutes and 600 mg infusion in 1 hour.

Adenosine is an increasingly popular drug for the treatment of these arrhythmias, but should not be given to patients with asthma or chronic obstructive airway disease. Cardioversion is often required if hypotension persists.

Sustained ventricular tachycardia must be treated promptly (see box 17.6). Again cardioversion is often required.

Box 17.6   Treatment of sustained ventricular tachycardia

(1) *If no hypotension*, but evidence of heart failure and heart rate <160 beats/ minute:

- give lignocaine 50 mg over 2 minutes, repeat every 5 minutes to a total dose of 200 mg; start infusion 2 mg/min
- check serum potassium
- give synchronised DC shock, 100 J, then 200 J, then 360 J
- give amiodarone 300 mg over 5–15 minutes then 600 mg over 1 hour
- give synchronised DC shock, 100 J, then 200 J, then 360 J.

(2) *If hypotension*, evidence of heart failure and heart rate >159 beats/minute:

- give synchronised DC shock, 100 J, then 200 J, then 360 J
- give 10 ml 50% magnesium sulphate in 1 hour
- give lignocaine as above
- perform further cardioversion as necessary
- for refractory cases consider:
  - procainamide
  - flecanide
  - bretylium *or*
  - overdrive pacing.

It should be noted that amiodarone may be used to treat both supraventricular and ventricular tachycardias.

Hypotension

Intraoperative hypotension is common and usually results from an inadequate blood volume following haemorrhage. The major causes are either a decreased venous return or a direct depression of the myocardium due to mechanical causes, myocardial disease, or anaesthetic drugs (Box 17.4).

Box 17.7 Major causes of intraoperative hypotension

- Decreased venous return:
  - *haemorrhage*
  - vena caval compression—obstetrics, prone position
  - drugs, infection

- Myocardial depression:
  - mechanical
    - intermittent positive pressure ventilation
    - equipment and circuit malfunction
    - pneumothorax
    - cardiac tamponade
    - pulmonary embolus
  - cardiac disease
  - drugs

Treatment is dependent on correct identification of the cause. Rapid intravenous infusion of colloid fluid or blood may be required, together with measurement of the central venous pressure. The use of inotropic drugs should only be considered when you are sure that there is an adequate circulating blood volume. Adrenaline is not an appropriate treatment for the hypotension of haemorrhage.

Laryngospasm

Reflex closure of the glottis from spasm of the vocal cords is due usually to laryngeal stimulation. Common causes include insertion of a Guedel airway or laryngoscope, the presence of a tracheal tube, and secretions in the airway. It can also arise as a response to surgical stimulation in a lightly anaesthetised patient. Thus, it occurs not only on induction of anaesthesia, but also intraoperatively, and occasionally postoperatively.

The airway obstruction can lead to hypoxia and, in severe cases, pulmonary oedema can result. The management of laryngospasm depends on its severity, as shown in box 17.8.

> **Box 17.8   Management of laryngospasm**
>
> (1) Identify stimulus and remove, if possible.
> (2) Give 100% O_2 and get help.
> (3) Ensure patent airway.
> (4) Tighten expiratory valve to apply a positive airway pressure to "break" the spasm and increase O_2 intake with each breath. (BE CAREFUL.)
> (5) If unable to ventilate, give suxamethonium, endotracheal intubation, and deepen anaesthesia. Ensure intubation and ventilation is feasible.

There is a belief that a patient with severe laryngospasm and cyanosis will gasp a breath just before hypoxaemia is fatal. Do not try to verify this tenet—if in doubt paralyse and ventilate the patient.

Wheeze

Wheeziness during anaesthesia may be caused by many factors other than bronchospasm (Box 17.5).

These causes must be eliminated before treatment for bronchospasm is started.

Complications associated with intubation often cause wheeze and it is essential to check the position and patency of the endotracheal tube first.

> **Box 17.9   Differential diagnoses of wheeze**
>
> - Oesophageal intubation
> - Tracheal tube in right main bronchus
> - Kinked tracheal tube
> - Tracheal tube cuff herniation over end of tube
> - Secretions in tracheal tube
> - Secretions in trachea/lungs
> - Gastric acid aspiration
> - Pneumothorax
> - Pulmonary oedema
> - Bronchospasm

Treatment of intraoperative bronchospasm is as follows:

(1) Consider changing volatile agent to halothane (bronchodilator).
(2) Give salbutamol 250 μg slowly i.v.
(3) Give aminophylline 250–500 mg (4–8 mg/kg) i.v. over 10–15 min.
(4) Give adrenaline 0·5–1·0 ml 1:10 000 increments i.v.
(5) Give hydrocortisone 100 mg i.v.

Conclusion

Many problems occur during the induction and maintenance of anaesthesia, and recovery of a patient. Whatever the problem, a cause must be sought in the following sequence: anaesthetic–surgical–medical. Only when the first two have been eliminated should specific medical therapy be started.

18: Postoperative problems

Intraoperative problems described in the previous chapter (arrhythmias, hypotension, laryngospasm, and wheeze) may continue, or even start, in the postoperative period. Investigation of the cause and subsequent management of these problems is identical, regardless of the time of onset.

Airway obstruction

Obstruction of the airway is a common occurrence after anaesthesia. It must be rapidly diagnosed (Box 18.1), the cause sought (Box 18.2), and appropriate treatment started.

> **Box 18.1 Signs of airway obstruction**
>
> - "See-saw" respiration pattern
> - Suprasternal and intercostal recession
> - Tachypnoea
> - Cyanosis
> - Tachycardia
> - Arrhythmias
> - Hypertension
> - Anxiety and distress
> - Sweating
> - Stridor

During emergence from anaesthesia patients may have incomplete mouth, pharyngeal, and laryngeal control, causing airway obstruction. Hypoxaemia will result if the airway is not maintained. Patients are turned routinely into the lateral or "recovery position" to help prevent this problem. The patient is usually placed in the left lateral position as reintubation is easier because laryngoscopes are designed to be inserted into the right side of the mouth.

If there is a possibility that aspiration may have occurred with the patient in the supine position, then they should be placed in the right lateral position to prevent contamination of the left lung.

Box 18.2 Common causes of postoperative airway obstruction

- Anaesthesia
  - unconsciousness with obstruction by tongue
  - laryngeal oedema
  - laryngeal spasm (Chapter 17).

- Surgery
  - vocal cord paralysis (thyroid surgery)
  - neck haematoma
  - preoperative neck and face inflammation (infection)

Patients who are at risk of aspiration should be extubated when the airway reflexes are intact. Although this is less pleasant for the patient, it is much safer.

The treatment of airway obstruction is to identify the cause, and clear the airway, often with suction, to ensure patency. Extension of the neck, jaw thrust, and insertion of an oropharyngeal airway, are often required. Laryngeal oedema is treated by intravenous dexamethosone 8 mg. Oxygenation of the patient is the priority and, if you are in doubt, reintubation must be undertaken. Many problems in anaesthesia are caused by inadequate attention to the airway. Remember, a patent airway is a happy airway.

Failure to breathe

Failure to breathe adequately at the end of anaesthesia has many causes, both common (Box 18.3) and unusual (Box 18.4).

Box 18.3 Common causes of failure to breathe

- Central nervous system
  - depression from drugs:
    - opiates
    - inhalational agents
  - decreased respiratory drive:
    - hypocapnia

- Peripheral
  - failure of neuromuscular transmission:
    - inadequate reversal of competitive relaxants
    - overdosage of competitive relaxants
    - cholinesterase deficiency

Box 18.4   Unusual causes of failure to breathe postoperatively

- Hypothermia
- Drug interactions:
  - aminoglycosides and competitive relaxants
  - ecothiopate and suxamethonium
- Central nervous system damage
- Electrolyte disorders:
  - hypokalaemia
- Undiagnosed skeletal muscle disorders:
  - myasthenia gravis
- Extensive spinal anaesthetic in combination with general anaesthesia

Differentiation between central and peripheral causes of failure to breathe can only be made by using a nerve stimulator. A peripheral nerve, such as the ulnar nerve at the wrist, is stimulated. Ensure that the nerve stimulator is working correctly; if necessary, try it on yourself first.

Adequate return of neuromuscular function is assessed by observing a "train of four" stimulation. Four twitches should be seen and the ratio of twitch four:twitch one response must exceed 70%. This is not easy to decide and we recommend that they should appear about equal. This ensures safety. A sustained tetanic response following high frequency stimulation also indicates adequate neuromuscular function (Box 18.5).

If a nerve stimulator is not available, there are clinical tests that can be made to indicate the return of normal neuromuscular activity.

Box 18.5   Signs of adequate neuromuscular function

- Evoked responses:
  - train of four ratio >70%
  - sustained tetanic response to high frequency stimulation
  - return of single twitch to control height

- Clinical responses:
  - lift head for 5 s
  - sustained hand grip
  - open eyes widely
  - sustained tongue protrusion
  - effective cough
  - adequate tidal volume
  - vital capacity 15–20 ml/kg

If inadequate neuromuscular function is found, the lungs must be ventilated and the use of neuromuscular blocking drugs reviewed.

Prolonged apnoea after suxamethonium occurs when the patient has an abnormal genetic variant of the plasma enzyme, cholinesterase. The patient and members of the family should be investigated at a later date and susceptible individuals asked to carry warning cards.

Only when you are certain that neuromuscular transmission is normal, should a central cause for failure to breathe be considered. Again the lungs must be ventilated, a normal end-tidal CO_2 concentration obtained and possible causes assessed (see box 18.3). An overdose of opioid is a common reason for failure to breathe. This can be treated with low doses of intravenous naloxone 40 µg, but this potent antagonist is short-acting and the return of adequate respiration is usually accompanied by a complete lack of analgesia! This is an unsatisfactory mess and it is better to ventilate the lungs until the central depressant effects of the drugs have worn off, or consider intravenous doxapram.

Box 18.6   Factors associated with postoperative vomiting

- Patient predisposition
  - age, sex, menstrual cycle, obesity
  - history of postoperative vomiting
  - history of motion sickness
  - anxiety, pain
  - recent food intake, prolonged fasting
- Surgical factors
  - type of surgery
  - emergency surgery
- Anaesthetic factors
  - inhalational agents
  - intravenous induction agents
  - opiates
  - duration of anaesthesia
  - distension of gut
  - oropharyngeal stimulation
  - experience of anaesthetist
- Postoperative factors
  - pain
  - hypotension
  - hypoxaemia
  - movement of patient
  - first intake of fluids/food
  - early mobilisation

Nausea and vomiting

Nausea and vomiting are particularly unpleasant complications of anaesthesia and surgery. The avoidance of these problems is more important to some patients than the provision of adequate analgesia. There are many factors associated with the occurrence of nausea and vomiting (Box 18.6). This long list indicates that often there is no single, identifiable cause, although opioids are frequently at fault.

Because patients find nausea and vomiting distressing, it should be prevented if possible. The medical consequences of vomiting include the possibility of acid aspiration, electrolyte imbalance and dehydration, inability to take oral drugs, and disruption of the wound. A vomiting patient upsets other patients in the recovery area and surgical ward. Most anaesthetists give antiemetics routinely. Drugs used include cyclizine, prochlorperazine, droperidol, metoclopramide, and ondansetron. The newer agents seem little better than traditional drugs.

Delayed awakening

Failure to recover full consciousness after surgery is always worrying for the anaesthetist. A systematic review of the patient is necessary (Box 18.7).

The most common causes are drug-related, but you must also remember the possibility of a low temperature, low blood glucose, low plasma sodium, and low circulating thyroid hormones.

Box 18.7   Causes of delayed recovery

- Hypoxaemia
- Hypercapnia
- Residual anaesthesia
- Drugs, especially opiates
- Emergence delirium from ketamine, scopolamine, atropine
- Neurological causes
- Surgery: neurosurgery, vascular surgery
- Metabolic causes:
  - hypoglycaemia
  - hyponatraemia
- Medical causes: hypothyroidism
- Sepsis
- Hypothermia

Shivering

Shivering is common during recovery from anaesthesia, but is not obviously related to a low core temperature in the patient. It is more frequent in young men who have received volatile agents and its incidence is decreased by the use of opiates during anaesthesia. The main deleterious effect of shivering is an increase in O_2 consumption. This is of little consequence in young, fit patients, but it should be treated promptly in the elderly who often have impaired cardiac and respiratory function.

Pethidine 25 mg intravenously is effective in stopping shivering; other opiates can also be used. Low doses of intravenous doxapram are an alternative to opiates if there is a risk of respiratory depression. The simple application of heat to the "blush area" (the face and upper chest) stops shivering. This indicates the importance of skin temperature in stimulating shivering as the effect on body temperature is negligible.

Temperature disturbances

A decrease in body temperature is an inevitable accompaniment of anaesthesia. Indeed, it has been noted that the most effective means of cooling a person is to give an anaesthetic. Hypothermia (defined as a core temperature <35°C), can occur after major surgery and the predisposing factors are shown in Box 18.8.

Box 18.8 Factors predisposing to postoperative hypothermia

- Ambient theatre temperature
- Age, young and elderly
- Surgery
  - duration
  - size of incision
  - insulation
- Concomitant disease
- Intravenous fluid administration
- Drug therapy such as vasodilators

Complications of postoperative hypothermia may include shivering (see above), impaired drug metabolism and enhanced platelet aggregation. There are several methods available for preventing loss of body heat during surgery (Box 18.9), and a combination of treatments is necessary. For example, the theatre temperature must be maintained at 24°C, the inspired gases humidified, the intravenous fluids warmed and the skin surface warmed.

> **Box 18.9   Prevention of body heat loss**
>
> - Ambient theatre temperature
> - Airway humidification
> - Warm skin surface
>   - passive insulation
>   - active warming
>   - water blanket
>   - radiant heater
>   - forced air warmer
> - Warm intravenous fluids
> - Oesophageal warming

Hyperthermia after anaesthesia is uncommon (Box 18.10). In the list below infection is the most common cause, and the potentially lethal complication of malignant hyperthermia should only be diagnosed after arterial gas analysis and determination of circulating potassium values (see Chapter 14).

> **Box 18.10   Causes of hyperthermia**
>
> - Infection
> - Environmental
> - Mismatched transfusion
> - Drugs
>   - interactions
>   - atropine overdose
> - Metabolic
>   - malignant hyperthermia
>   - phaeochromocytoma
>   - hyperthyroidism

Cyanosis

Cyanosis is a serious sequelae of anaesthesia and, whenever it occurs, must be investigated promptly:

(1) Check oxygen delivery from anaesthetic machine and circuit.
(2) Check airway. Is endotracheal tube correctly positioned and patent?
(3) Having excluded these causes, consider:
  - fault in chest (is ventilation easy?):
    - bronchospasm
    - pulmonary oedema

- pneumothorax
- pulmonary effusion/haemothorax.
- fault in circulation:
  - decreased venous return
  - cardiac failure
  - embolism
  - drug reaction.

(4) Rare causes include:
  - methaemoglobinaemia
  - malignant hyperthermia.

Problems of the airway are the most common causes of cyanosis and you must be *certain* that the airway is patent and the patient is breathing O_2 before considering other causes.

Conclusion

Postoperative problems often reflect errors of judgement made during surgery. Get it right intraoperatively and your patients will have fewer difficulties postoperatively. Nursing staff in the recovery area and surgical wards rapidly assess your anaesthetic skills by the smoothness of recovery of your patients.

Part III
Passing the gas

As the weeks of your anaesthetic career become months, you will play an increasing part in the preoperative assessment of patients and the conduct of the anaesthetic. In this section of the book we describe briefly the anaesthetic considerations of some of the common surgical specialties with which a trainee is often involved. We have deliberately excluded any pharmacology of the anaesthetic drugs. There is no evidence to show any benefit from a particular anaesthetic technique in terms of postoperative morbidity and mortality. The principles of anaesthesia are more important than the choice of drugs.

The key feature of this section is the need for a thorough preoperative evaluation of all patients. This is the cornerstone of safe anaesthetic practice and must *never* be omitted.

19: Preoperative evaluation

Preoperative evaluation is used to assess the anaesthetic risks in relation to the proposed surgery, to decide the anaesthetic technique (general, regional, or a combination), and to plan the postoperative care including any analgesic regimens. Explanation of the relevant details of the anaesthetic can be given, and the use of premedication can be discussed. Patients waiting for surgery are vulnerable and a friendly, professional approach by the anaesthetist is essential.

Operations are classified into 4 groups (Box 19.1).

Box 19.1   Classification of operations

- Emergency: immediate operation within one hour of surgical consultation and considered life-saving, for example, ruptured aortic aneurysm repair.

- Urgent: operation as soon as possible after resuscitation, usually within 24 hours of surgical consultation, for example, intestinal obstruction.

- Scheduled: early operation between 1 and 3 weeks, which is not immediately life-saving, for example, cancer surgery, cardiac surgery.

- Elective: operation at a time to suit both the patient and surgeon.

This classification has been agreed with the surgeons, but their memory often fails, so do not be surprised to find elective cases suddenly classified as emergencies. This is usually done for surgical convenience.

It is sometimes difficult to convey an overall impression of the complexity of a patient's medical condition and this can be done by referring to one of the five American Society of Anesthesiologists (ASA) Physical Status Classes (Box 19.2). It is important to remember that this only refers to the physical status of the patient and does not consider other relevant factors such as age, and nature and duration of surgery.

Preoperative assessment is outlined below.

(1) History
- age
- present illness

- drugs
- allergies
- past history (operations and anaesthetics)
- anaesthetic family history
- social (smoking, alcohol)

(2) Examination
- AIRWAY (see Chapter 1)
- teeth
- general examination

(3) Specific assessment

(4) Investigations

(5) Consent

(6) Premedication.

Box 19.2   ASA physical status classes

- ASA1:   normal healthy patient.

- ASA2:   patient with mild controlled systemic disease which does not affect normal activity, for example, mild diabetes, mild hypertension.

- ASA3:   patient with severe systemic disease which limits activity, for example, angina, chronic bronchitis.

- ASA4:   patient with incapacitating systemic disease that is a constant threat to life.

- ASA5:   moribund patient not expected to survive 24 hours either with or without an operation.

- E: emergency procedure.

The history of the present illness is important. For example, in orthopaedic surgery, a fractured neck of femur may occur for many reasons: a fall from an accident, stroke, cardiac episode (Stokes–Adams attack) or a spontaneous fracture from a metastasis.

The subsequent examination and investigations are obviously different in each case. Drug therapy is usually continued throughout the operative period (especially cardiac drugs and antihypertensive agents). Potential drug interactions should be sought. Details of any previous anaesthetics may indicate difficulties with endotracheal intubation. Unfortunately successful intubation in the past is no guarantee of future success. A family history of cholinesterase deficiency and malignant hyperthermia should be sought.

A specific assessment of the concurrent disease(s) must also be undertaken. The specific problem of obesity is evaluated as shown in Box 19.3.

Box 19.3   Specific assessment of obesity

- Psychological aspects
- Drug metabolism
- Associated diseases
  - hypertension
  - coronary artery disease
  - diabetes
- Difficult venous access
- Airway
  - difficult to intubate
  - difficult to maintain
- Hypoxaemia more likely intraoperatively—ventilation mandatory
- Regional anaesthesia—difficult to perform
- Position of patient for surgery
- Postoperative analgesia and physiotherapy to decrease chest complications
- Immobility and deep vein thrombosis—prophylaxis
- Wound dehiscence and wound infection

Only appropriate investigations should be undertaken. A typical list of basic tests is shown in Box 19.4.

Box 19.4   Basic preoperative tests

- Haemoglobin concentration
- Screening for sickle cell disease
- Blood urea, creatinine and electrolyte concentrations
- Blood glucose
- Chest X-ray
- ECG

A lot of money is wasted on unnecessary preoperative tests. When you have taken a history from the patient and conducted the relevant examination, you must then decide what tests, if any, are required. A young, fit sportsman for an arthroscopy requires no further investigation; whereas an elderly West Indian patient who has diabetes, hypertension, coronary artery disease, and needs major vascular surgery, requires all the tests listed in Box 19.4 and probably more. In many hospitals there are guidelines on the use of preoperative investigations. These can be helpful, as they reflect local practice. For example, you may find that there is far greater use of preoperative chest X-rays in regions with a high population of recent immigrants to exclude tuberculosis.

On completion of the preoperative assessment, and with the results of the relevant investigations available, a plan for the anaesthetic care of the patient can be decided. The following surgical factors must also be considered.

- When is the operation to occur?
- Who is operating?
- Where is the patient going postoperatively (home, ward, HDU, ITU)?

Occasionally it is necessary to postpone surgery. This is most often done on medical grounds, for example to improve cardiac failure, treat arrhythmias, control blood pressure. In the early months of your anaesthetic career, seek senior advice before postponing surgery; this prevents prolonged arguments with surgical colleagues.

Premedication

The use of premedication is declining, although most anaesthetists undergoing surgery demand heavy sedation. The wishes of the patient must be considered. The main reasons for giving premedication are shown in Box 19.5.

Box 19.5   Reasons for premedication

- Anxiolysis
- Antisialogue
- Analgesia
- Antiemesis
- Amnesia
- Decreased gastric acidity
- Part of anaesthetic technique (assist induction)
- Prevention of unwanted vagal responses
- Prevention of needle pain

A variety of drugs including opiates, benzodiazepines, anticholinergics, phenothiazines, and H_2 receptor blocking drugs are used. It is important to remember that opiates may make patients vomit. Topical EMLA cream can be used to prevent the pain of insertion of a cannula. This eutectic mixture of prilocaine and lignocaine (1 g of EMLA contains 25 mg of each) is applied to the dorsum of the hands for a minimum of 1 h to a maximum of 5 h before induction of anaesthesia.

Conclusion

Preoperative assessment is often difficult and its importance should not be underestimated. The anaesthetic care of the patient can only be planned after a thorough assessment, together with the results of relevant investigations, and precise knowledge of the proposed surgery.

20: Regional anaesthesia

Local anaesthetic agents are used to provide intraoperative analgesia, either as the sole anaesthetic technique or in combination with sedation or general anaesthesia. You should learn the principles of regional anaesthesia at an early stage of your training.

The drugs in common use are lignocaine, bupivacaine, and prilocaine and their characteristics are shown in Box 20.1. The choice of drug depends on the speed of onset and duration of action required. Adrenaline prolongs the latter.

Box 20.1 Characteristics of local anaesthetic drugs			
Agent	Duration (h)	Maximum dose	
		plain (mg/kg)	with adrenaline (mg/kg)
Lignocaine	1–3	3	7
Bupivacaine	1–4	2	2
Prilocaine	1–3	4	8

Local anaesthetic drugs have serious side effects if given in excess, or inadvertently into the circulation. Toxicity is manifest in a variety of ways ranging from mild excitation to serious neurological and fatal cardiac sequelae (Box 20.2).

Box 20.2 Symptoms and signs of local anaesthetic toxicity

- Anxiety
- Restlessness
- Nausea
- Tinnitus
- Circumoral tingling
- Tremor
- Tachypnoea
- Clonic convulsions
- Arrhythmias
  - ventricular fibrillation
  - asystole

Adrenaline is sometimes added to the local anaesthetic to prolong its action, and to decrease the vascularity of an operative field (for example, in thyroid surgery). It must not be used near terminal arterioles or arteries, as an adequate collateral arterial supply is not available to perfuse distal tissues, and ischaemia will occur. The recommendations for the safe use of adrenaline are listed in Box 20.3.

Box 20.3 Recommendations for the safe use of adrenaline in local anaesthetic solutions

- No hypoxia
- No hypercapnia
- Caution with arrhythmogenic volatile agents, for example, halothane
- Concentration of $\leq 1:200\,000$
- Dose <20 ml of 1:200 000 in 10 min
- Total dose <30 ml/hour

Occasionally the anaesthetist is responsible for supervising the preparation of a 1:200 000 adrenaline solution. The commonly available dilutions of adrenaline are 1:10 000 and 1 in 1000. Therefore, either:

1 ml of 1:10 000 adrenaline diluted to a total volume of 20 ml = 1:200 000 solution *or*

0·1 ml of 1:1000 adrenaline diluted to a total volume of 20 ml = 1:200 000 solution.

The former is more accurate, as measuring 0·1 ml exactly is not easy. A similar calculation to that described in Chapter 11, shows that 1 ml of 1:200 000 adrenaline solution contains 5 µg adrenaline.

Before undertaking regional anaesthesia, the following criteria must be considered and satisfied (Box 20.4).

Box 20.4   Requirements before starting regional anaesthesia

- Informed consent
- Vascular access
- Resuscitation drugs and equipment
- Sterility of anaesthetist
- Sterility of operative site
- No contraindications to procedure
- Correct dosage of local anaesthetic drug

Sterility of the anaesthetist does not refer to their reproductive capacity, but means wearing a gown, mask, hat, and gloves.

Epidural anaesthesia

The epidural space runs from the base of the skull to the bottom of the sacrum at the sacrococcygeal membrane. The spinal cord, cerebrospinal fluid, and meninges are enclosed within it (Figure 20.1).

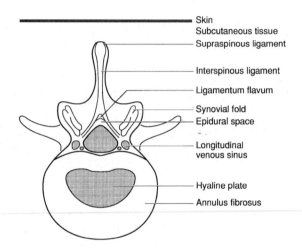

Skin
Subcutaneous tissue
Supraspinous ligament

Interspinous ligament

Ligamentum flavum

Synovial fold
Epidural space

Longitudinal
venous sinus

Hyaline plate

Annulus fibrosus

FIG 20.1—*Anatomy of the epidural space*

The spinal cord becomes the cauda equina at the level of L2 in an adult and the cerebrospinal fluid stops at the level of S2. The epidural space is between 3–6 mm wide and is defined posteriorly by the ligamentum flavum, the anterior surfaces of the vertebral laminae, and the articular processes. Anteriorly it is related to the posterior longitudinal ligament and laterally is bounded by the intervertebral foramenae and the pedicles.

The contents of the epidural space are:

- nerve roots
- venous plexus
- fat
- lymphatics.

The veins contain no valves and communicate directly with the intracranial, thoracic, and abdominal venous systems.

Contraindications to epidural anaesthesia are shown in Box 20.5. Abnormal clotting may result in haemorrhage in a confined space if an epidural vein is punctured during the insertion of an epidural cannula. An epidural haematoma then causes spinal cord compression. Local skin infection may introduce bacteria into the spinal meninges with the risk of an abscess or meningitis. Similarly in septicaemia, if a vein is punctured then the small haematoma is a good culture medium for bacteria.

Box 20.5   Absolute and relative contraindications to epidural anaesthesia

- Absolute
  - patient refusal
  - abnormal clotting
  - infection—local on back, septicaemia
  - allergy to local anaesthetic drug

- Relative
  - raised intracranial pressure
  - hypovolaemia
  - chronic spinal disorders
  - central nervous system disease
  - drugs—aspirin, other NSAIDs, low dose heparin

Although the evidence that spinal disorders are exacerbated by the insertion of an epidural catheter is poor, patients are often quick to blame the anaesthetic procedure. The same principle applies to patients with neurological problems such as multiple sclerosis. The evidence that drugs which mildly affect clotting or platelet function (for example, non-steroidal anti-inflammatory drugs) cause abnormal bleeding in the epidural space and increase the risk of an epidural haematoma is minimal.

The equipment used for the insertion of an epidural catheter is shown in Figure 20.2.

The Tuohy needle is either 16 or 18 gauge. It is 10 cm long: 8 cm of needle and 2 cm of hub. It is marked in centimetres and has a curved "Huber" tip. The epidural catheter has three holes at 120° alignment with the holes 2 cm from the end of the catheter. The catheter is marked in centimetre gradations up to 20 cm. The filter has a 0·2 μm mesh which stops the injection of particulate matter, such as glass, and bacteria into the epidural space.

The correct technique of insertion of an epidural catheter must be learnt under careful supervision. The conditions listed in Box 20.3 must be met. An intravenous infusion of either crystalloid or colloid is set up to give a "fluid load" of about 500 ml before the local anaesthetic is injected. This is undertaken to decrease the likelihood of hypotension with the onset of the epidural block. Atropine and a vasopressor should always be drawn up before starting the block.

The procedure can be done in either the lateral or sitting position and ideally the spine should be flexed. A slow, controlled advance of the Tuohy needle is essential, using a syringe and a loss of resistance technique. The needle passes through skin, subcutaneous tissue, supraspinous ligament, interspinous ligament, ligamentum flavum, and finally enters the epidural

105

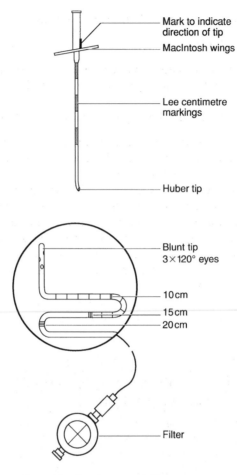

FIG 20.2—*Tuohy needle, epidural catheter, and filter*

space. The ligaments resist the injection of air or saline, but when the needle enters the epidural space the resistance is lost.

The choice is between using air or saline to identify the epidural space. The *advantages of air* are that:

- any fluid in the needle or catheter must be cerebrospinal fluid;
- there is less equipment on the tray;
- it is cheaper.

The *disadvantages of air* are that:

- injection of large volumes may result in patchy blockade;
- there is a theoretical risk of air embolus.

The *advantages of saline* are that:

- it is a more reliable method of identifying the epidural space;

106

- the catheter passes more easily into epidural space.

The *disadvantages of saline* are that:

- fluid in the needle or catheter, may be saline or cerebrospinal fluid; the latter is warmer and contains glucose but rapid clinical decisions are difficult;
- there is additional fluid on the tray with increased risk of error.

We recommend you become thoroughly familiar with either air or saline before trying the alternative method. There is no "correct" method; one author uses air and the other uses saline.

The epidural space is usually found at a distance of about 4–6 cm from the skin. Place the catheter rostrally and, using the centimetre markings on the needle and catheter, insert 3 cm of catheter into the epidural space.

The filter and catheter, once correctly positioned and fixed, must be aspirated to ensure that no blood or cerebrospinal fluid can be withdrawn. The local anaesthetic drug is given in small, incremental doses to reduce the risk of complications.

The complications of epidural blockade, assuming no technical difficulties in the location of the space and the siting of the catheter, are shown in Boxes 20.6 and 20.7.

Box 20.6   Major complications of epidural analgesia

- Severe hypotension
- Accidental intravenous injection
- Dural puncture
  - massive spinal anaesthetic
  - headache

Hypotension results from a decreased venous return to the heart as a consequence of vasodilation induced by the sympathetic blockade. The "fluid load" helps to prevent hypotension, but a vasoconstrictor, such as ephedrine in 3–6 mg intravenous increments, is often given to restore normal arterial pressure.

The risks of the intravenous injection of local anaesthetic are minimised by aspiration of the cannula and by giving small incremental doses. If blood is aspirated, usually the cannula is removed and the epidural resited in a different space. Occasionally the cannula can be withdrawn from the epidural vein and no blood aspirated. Then the epidural catheter must be flushed with saline to ensure the cannula is not in a vein before further use.

Accidental, dural puncture occurs when the needle or cannula is inserted into the cerebrospinal fluid. If this is not recognised and a full epidural

107

dose of local anaesthetic is injected into the wrong place, a massive spinal anaesthetic will result with apnoea, severe hypotension, and total paralysis. The lungs have to be ventilated and the circulation supported during this period. For this reason an epidural "test dose" of 2–3 ml of local anaesthetic is given by many anaesthetists before the full dose is injected (for example, 2% lignocaine). In the epidural space this dose of local anaesthetic has little effect, but in the cerebrospinal fluid an extensive block occurs rapidly. After 10 min the epidural dose of local anaesthetic is given if no adverse effects are noted.

A severe postural headache following dural puncture is managed by resting the patient in a flat position, simple analgesics, adequate hydration, caffeine and, if necessary, a "blood patch". The dural puncture can be sealed by placing 20 ml of the patient's blood into the epidural space under aseptic conditions. The resulting clot will rapidly stop the leak and is effective in virtually all patients. Two anaesthetists are required for this manoeuvre.

Box 20.7   Other complications of epidural analgesia

- Leg weakness
- Shivering
- Atonic bladder
- Contraction of the small bowel
- Backache
- Isolated, reversible nerve damage from catheter/needle trauma
- Epidural haematoma
- Epidural abscess
- Meningitis

Opiates can also be given in the epidural space to prolong the effects of local anaesthetics and to provide postoperative analgesia. They have different complications (Box 20.8) of which respiratory depression is the most serious. Regular monitoring of respiratory function is essential (see Chapter 28).

Box 20.8   Complications of epidural opiates

- Delayed respiratory depression
- Drowsiness
- Itchiness
- Nausea and vomiting
- Urinary retention

108

Spinal anaesthesia

This is the deliberate injection of local anaesthetic into the cerebrospinal fluid (CSF) by means of a lumbar puncture. It is normally given as a single injection, but can be used in conjunction with epidural anaesthesia (combined spinal–epidural anaesthesia) for longer procedures. The incidence of headache following dural puncture is dependent on the size and type of spinal needle. Not surprisingly, the smaller the diameter of the needle, the lower the incidence of headache (remember 27 gauge is *smaller* than 25 gauge).

Pencil-tip, spinal needles, such as Whiteacre and Sprotte, split, rather than cut, the dura and also reduce the risk of headache.

Local anaesthetic solutions for spinal anaesthesia are isobaric or hyperbaric with respect to the CSF. Isobaric solutions are claimed to have a more predictable spread in the CSF, independent of the position of the patient. Hyperbaric solutions are produced by the addition of glucose and their spread is partially influenced by gravity. Many factors determine the distribution of local anaesthetic solutions in the CSF; this makes prediction of the level of blockade difficult (Box 20.9).

> **Box 20.9   Factors influencing distribution of local anaesthetic solutions in CSF**
>
> - Local anaesthetic drug
> - Baricity
> - Dose of drug
> - Volume of drug
> - Turbulence of cerebrospinal fluid
> - Increased abdominal pressure
> - Spinal curvatures
> - Position of patient
> - Use of vasoconstrictors
> - Speed of injection

The complications of spinal anaesthesia are the same as for epidural anaesthesia. Neuronal blockade is more rapid in onset so that the side effects, such as hypotension, occur promptly. In spinal anaesthesia the duration of the block is variable but is usually shorter than that of epidural analgesia.

Caudal anaesthesia

The caudal space is a continuation of the epidural space in the sacral region. The signet-shaped, sacral hiatus is formed by the failure of fusion of the laminae of the 5th sacral vertebra. The hiatus is bounded laterally by the sacral cornua and is covered by the posterior sacrococcygeal ligament, subcutaneous tissue, and skin. The epidural space is located by passing a needle through the sacral hiatus. The caudal canal contains veins, fat, and the sacral nerves. The cerebrospinal fluid finishes at the level of S2.

Caudal anaesthesia is used for operations in areas supplied by the sacral nerves, such as anal surgery and circumcision. The precautions are the same as those described for epidural analgesia. The needle must be aspirated after insertion to exclude blood and cerebrospinal fluid. The complications are the same as for epidural anaesthesia, although motor blockade can be a major problem in the early postoperative period if the patient wants to walk.

Hypotension is uncommon, as the neuronal blockade usually does not spread rostrally to reach the sympathetic chain.

The extent of a block can be measured by the absence of pain or temperature sensation at a dermatomal level (Box 20.10). The former is tested with a sharp needle and the latter with an ethyl chloride spray.

Box 20.10 Dermatomal levels at various anatomical landmarks

Anatomical landmark	Dermatological levels
Nipples	T4
Xiphisternum	T6
Umbilicus	T10
Symphysis pubis	L1/T12

Intravenous regional analgesia

A limb can be anaesthetised by the administration of local anaesthetic intravenously distal to a tourniquet placed high on the limb. This technique is used on the arm only, because the leg needs toxic doses of local anaesthetics. It is used commonly for manipulation of fractures and brief operations on the hand. The precautions mentioned in Box 20.3 must be adhered to.

An intravenous cannula is inserted into a vein on the dorsum of the hand. A single or double cuff is placed around the humerus. If a double cuff is used, the higher cuff is compressed first until the arm is anaesthetised, and then the lower cuff is inflated over the numb skin to make it more comfortable for the patient. The cuff is pressurised to 250–300 mm Hg and about 40 ml 0·5% prilocaine without adrenaline (see Table 20.1) injected into the arm. The patient will often only tolerate the cuff for 45–60 min because of pain. The cuff must remain inflated for at least

20 min, otherwise systemic toxicity may occur from rapid uptake of the drug when the tourniquet is released.

The main problem with this block is the tourniquet. It must not deflate accidentally.

Conclusion

Regional anaesthesia is fun for the anaesthetist and provides excellent analgesia for the patient. The successful use of these techniques depends on learning good technical skills to match understanding of essential anatomy, physiology, and pharmacology. Start early in your career—make the epidural space a familiar territory.

21: Principles of emergency anaesthesia

In elective surgery the correct diagnosis has been made (usually), any medical disorders have been identified and treated, and an appropriate period of starvation has occurred. During emergency work, however, one or more of these conditions are often not met. In addition, there are further problems such as:

- dehydration
- electrolyte abnormalities
- haemorrhage
- pain.

The components of general anaesthesia are the same, whether it is conducted for elective surgery or emergency surgery (Box 21.1).

> **Box 21.1   Components of general anaesthesia**
>
> - Preoperative assessment
> - Premedication
> - Induction
> - Maintenance
> - Reversal
> - Postoperative care

The key to success in emergency anaesthesia is a thorough preoperative assessment. It should be undertaken as described in Chapter 19. Particular attention must be given to the search for medical problems, the occurrence of hypovolaemia, and an evaluation of the airway. On the basis of the preoperative, clinical assessment together with the results of *relevant* investigations, then a decision can be reached about an appropriate time to operate.

There are very few patients whose clinical state is so life-threatening that they need immediate surgery, i.e. a true "emergency" (see Box 19.1). The vast majority of patients benefit greatly from the correction of hypovolaemia and electrolyte abnormalities, stabilisation of medical problems such as diabetes and cardiac arrhythmias, and waiting for the stomach to empty.

If necessary, preoperative optimisation should be undertaken in ITU. Surgeons are not known for their patience and often view any delay in operating as time wasted. *When to operate* is the most important decision that has to be made in emergency work. Fortunately for the patient, and for you, it is made increasingly by senior staff. In the early stages of your anaesthetic career you should observe closely the evidence used to reach that decision.

Although it is usually assumed that emergency anaesthesia means general anaesthesia, other methods can sometimes be employed (Box 21.2).

Box 21.2   Classification of anaesthetic techniques

- General anaesthesia
  - intubation of unprotected airway
  - spontaneous respiration or controlled ventilation
  - use of muscle relaxants
- Regional anaesthesia
- Combination of general and regional anaesthesia
- Sedation
  - intravenous
  - inhalational
- Combination of sedation and regional anaesthesia

There is increasing use of regional anaesthesia, but hypovolaemia must be corrected preoperatively. Sedation should not be confused with general anaesthesia. The sedated patient can talk to the anaesthetist at all times. If not, then airway control may be lost with the risk of aspiration of gastric contents.

Full stomach

Patients for elective surgery are usually starved for 4–6 hours to ensure an empty stomach, but can receive clear fluids for up to 2 hours before induction of anaesthesia. Nevertheless, every few years we have the unpleasant experience of dealing with elective patients who vomit undigested food at least 12 hours after the meal in the absence of any intestinal abnormalities. In emergency surgery it is usual to starve the patient for at least 4–6 hours. However, this rule is unreliable and all emergency patients should be treated as having a full stomach and so at risk of vomiting, regurgitation and aspiration.

Vomiting occurs at the induction of, and emergence from, anaesthesia. If gastric acid enters the lungs a pneumonitis results which can be fatal. Aspiration can also occur following passive regurgitation of gastric contents up the oesophagus. This regurgitation is often described as "silent" to distinguish it from active vomiting. Regurgitation is particularly likely at induction of anaesthesia when several drugs used (atropine, thiopentone, suxamethonium) decrease the pressure in the lower oesophageal sphincter.

In emergency anaesthesia there is always a risk of aspiration, regardless of the period of starvation. Therefore, the trachea must be intubated as rapidly as possible after induction of anaesthesia. The methods available are shown in Box 21.3. If preoperative assessment of the airway indicates no problems then endotracheal intubation is performed under general anaesthesia. However, *if a difficult airway is predicted then senior help must be called.*

Box 21.3   Methods of facilitating tracheal intubation

- Patient awake
  - topical anaesthesia

- Patient anaesthetised
  - use of muscle relaxants
    - suxamethonium
    - competitive relaxants
  - inhalational techniques

There are some basic requirements for endotracheal intubation in emergency surgery:

- skilled assistance must be present;
- the trolley must tip;
- the suction apparatus must work correctly and is left on;
- a range of sizes of endotracheal tubes must be available;
- spare laryngoscopes must be available;
- ancillary intubation aids, gum elastic bougie, stillettes, etc. must be available.

A plan of management of the patient who may have a full stomach and is at risk of aspiration is shown in Box 21.4.

Neither physical nor pharmacological methods should be relied on to empty the stomach completely. In some specialties such as obstetrics, an H_2 receptor blocking drug, ranitidine, is given routinely to decrease gastric acid secretion and 30 ml sodium citrate used orally 15 min before induction of anaesthesia to increase the pH of the gastric contents. Opiates delay gastric emptying and increase the likelihood of vomiting.

The only reliable way to prevent regurgitation is to use the correct anaesthetic technique. This is now called a rapid sequence induction which

> ## Box 21.4 Management of endotracheal intubation when risk of aspiration
>
> - Empty stomach
>   - from above by nasogastric tube
>   - from below by drugs, for example, metoclopramide
> - Neutralise remaining stomach contents
>   - antacids
>   - use of H_2 blocking drugs to prevent further acid secretion
> - Stop central nervous system induced vomiting
>   - avoid opiates
>   - use of phenothiazines
> - CORRECT ANAESTHETIC TECHNIQUE
>   - "rapid sequence induction"
>   - preoxygenation, cricoid pressure, intubation

sounds better than the old term—crash induction. It has three essential components: preoxygenation, cricoid pressure, intubation.

Preoxygenation

Before induction the patient must breathe 100% oxygen for at least 3 min from a suitable breathing circuit. There should be no leaks and the flow rate of oxygen in the circuit should be high to prevent rebreathing. Air contains oxygen, nitrogen, and minimal carbon dioxide. When the patient is breathing oxygen only, the lungs denitrogenate rapidly and after 3 min contain only oxygen and carbon dioxide. There is now a greater reservoir of oxygen in the lungs to utilise before hypoxia occurs.

Anaesthesia is then induced and cricoid pressure applied.

Cricoid pressure

The cricoid cartilage is identified on the patient before anaesthesia is induced and the patient warned that they might feel pressure on the neck as they go to sleep. The skilled assistant presses down on the cricoid cartilage as anaesthesia is induced and *this pressure is applied continuously until the anaesthetist tells the assistant to stop* (Figure 21.1).

The object of pressure on the cricoid cartilage is to compress the oesophagus between the cricoid cartilage and vertebral column. This prevents any material that has been regurgitated from the stomach into the oesophagus from passing into the pharynx.

Cricoid pressure is usually undertaken by firm, but gentle, pressure on the cartilage by the thumb and forefinger of the assistant. It is similar to the pressure exerted that causes mild pain when the thumb and forefinger

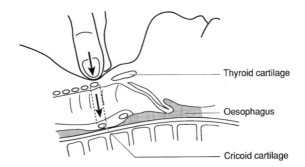

FIG 21.1—*Application of cricoid pressure*

are pressed onto the bridge of the nose. The cricoid cartilage is used because it is easily identifiable, forms a complete tracheal ring, and the trachea is not distorted when it is compressed.

The patient has now received preoxygenation, an induction agent, and cricoid pressure. A neuromuscular blocking drug is given to facilitate intubation of the trachea.

Intubation

The neuromuscular blocking drug must act rapidly and have a short duration of action. The lungs are *not* ventilated during a rapid sequence induction; this will prevent accidental inflation of the stomach which will further predispose the patient to regurgitation and vomiting. Gases can be forced into the oesophagus and stomach during manual ventilation of the lungs despite the application of cricoid pressure.

A drug with a rapid onset of action permits quick endotracheal intubation. An agent with a short duration of action is valuable because in cases of failed intubation spontaneous respiration will return promptly. This allows other options to be considered (Chapter 4).

Suxamethonium has many side effects (Box 21.5) but remains the best drug available.

Box 21.5   Major side effects of suxamethonium

- Muscle aches
- Bradycardia
- Raised intracranial pressure
- Raised intraocular pressure
- Raised intragastric pressure
- Allergic reactions
- Hyperkalaemia in burns, paraplegia, some myopathies
- Prolonged action in pseudocholinesterase deficiency
- Malignant hyperthermia

116

Only when the trachea is intubated, the cuff inflated and the correct position of the tube confirmed, is the cricoid pressure released.

The anaesthetic is maintained, usually with a volatile agent, nitrous oxide, oxygen, competitive relaxant, and suitable analgesia. The reversal of the relaxant at the end of the procedure is undertaken with the anticholinesterase, neostigmine. Atropine or glycopyrrolate is given concomitantly to stop bradycardia occurring from the neostigmine.

Rapid sequence induction has the major disadvantage of potential haemodynamic instability, as hypertension and tachycardia often occur following laryngoscopy and intubation. This is often more severe than in elective surgery when opiates are often given at induction of anaesthesia.

Other indications for rapid sequence induction

Every anaesthetic, not just emergency work, should be considered from the point of view of unexpected vomiting or regurgitation. Some cases are at high risk and rapid sequence induction should be considered carefully as an option in this group (Box 21.6).

Box 21.6   Factors in high risk of regurgitation

- Oesophageal disease
  - pouch
  - stricture

- Gastro-oesophageal sphincter abnormalities
  - hiatus hernia
  - obesity
  - drugs

- Gastric emptying delay
  - trauma
  - pyloric stenosis
  - gastric malignancy
  - opiates
  - patient predisposition, anxiety
  - pregnancy
  - recent food intake

- Abnormal bowel peristalsis
  - peritonitis
  - ileus—metabolic or drugs
  - bowel obstruction

Pulmonary aspiration

Pulmonary aspiration may be obvious. The presence of lager and curry in the pharynx when the blade of the laryngoscope is inserted is a depressing sight. It may also be silent, presenting as a postoperative pulmonary complication.

The signs of pulmonary aspiration are shown in Box 21.7.

> ### Box 21.7 Signs of pulmonary aspiration
>
> - None
> - Oxygen desaturation
> - Coughing
> - Tachypnoea
> - Unexplained tachycardia
> - Wheeze
> - Hypotension
> - Pneumonitis
> - Postoperative pulmonary disease

Treatment requires the advice of a senior anaesthetist. The airway must be suctioned and *oxygenation of the patient remains the priority*. Bronchoscopy may be required to remove particulate matter. If the patient is not paralysed then, surgery permitting, he or she should be allowed to wake up. If paralysed, intubation and ventilation must occur and oxygenation maintained. Wheeze may be treated with aminophylline. Further treatment includes antibiotics, other bronchodilators, and steroids. Aggressive early management is required.

Conclusion

Anaesthesia for emergency surgery needs careful preoperative assessment and adequate resuscitation must be undertaken before surgery. Impatient surgeons must be restrained. A rapid sequence induction of anaesthesia must follow the order of preoxygenation, cricoid pressure and intubation to prevent aspiration of gastric contents.

22: Anaesthesia for gynaecological surgery

Gynaecological surgery is undertaken for diagnostic and therapeutic reasons. The trainee anaesthetist is often introduced to anaesthesia by means of supervised teaching on routine gynaecology lists. Laparoscopic procedures are increasingly common in gynaecological surgery.

Laparoscopy

Laparoscopy requires the formation of a pneumoperitoneum, and carbon dioxide is used as the insufflating gas for reasons shown in Box 22.1.

Box 22.1   Advantages of CO_2 use in pneumoperitoneum formation

- Cheap
- Readily available
- Nontoxic
- Does not support combustion
- More soluble in blood than air (20 ×)
- Buffered by formation of bicarbonate
- Easily excreted by the lungs

There are three main anaesthetic considerations when surgery is conducted laparoscopically:

- problems from gas insufflation;
- trauma by Verres needle or trochar;
- anaesthetic complications.

Problems from gas insufflation (Box 22.2)

When carbon dioxide is insufflated to cause the pneumoperitoneum, certain physiological changes occur in the cardiovascular and respiratory systems.

119

> ## Box 22.2 Problems arising from gas insufflation
>
> - Cardiovascular changes
> - Respiratory changes
> - Cardiac arrhythmias
> - Misplacement of the insufflating gas
> - Gas embolism
> - Hypothermia

Insufflation pressures of 10–15 mm Hg are well tolerated but pressures greater than 30 mm Hg can result in profound haemodynamic responses. The pneumoperitoneum increases intra-abdominal and intrathoracic pressures. This decreases venous return and so lowers cardiac output. In contrast, carbon dioxide absorption increases sympathetic activity to augment cardiac contractility and increase heart rate. During anaesthesia there is usually a satisfactory circulation with a normal or raised arterial blood pressure and a tachycardia. Problems arise, however, when haemorrhage occurs, as the usual compensatory cardiovascular responses may be inadequate.

Diaphragmatic splinting can result in basal atelectasis, increased intrapulmonary shunts, hypoxia, and hypercarbia in spontaneously breathing patients. These changes are minimised by positive pressure ventilation.

Cardiac arrhythmias may result from a low cardiac output in the presence of hypercarbia.

Inadvertent misplacement of the insufflating gas can cause subcutaneous emphysema, pneumomediastinum, pneumothorax, and pneumo-pericardium. Although rare, we have seen all these complications, with the exception of a pneumopericardium.

Carbon dioxide gas embolism is a major complication, as a large embolus will cause outflow obstruction of the pulmonary artery. The diagnosis is made by the occurrence of sudden hypotension, hypoxia, and a low expired carbon dioxide tension.

Hypothermia may occur in long procedures. A 0·3°C decrease in core temperature has been found for each 50 l of carbon dioxide insufflated.

Trauma by Verres needle or trochar

Major damage can occur (Box 22.3).

> ## Box 22.3 Complications from needle or trochar insertion
>
> - Haemorrhage
> - Intestinal perforation
> - Other visceral trauma

Haemorrhage can result from the passage of the trochar or needle through the anterior abdominal wall. Tearing of adhesions from the expanding pneumoperitoneum will also cause bleeding. Traumatic puncture of the major intra-abdominal vessels has been reported. One author observed a large tear in the internal iliac artery, which was ultimately fatal. The raised intra-abdominal pressure may tamponade even a large vessel and venous haemorrhage may not be obvious during the laparoscopy leading to a delay in a subsequent laparotomy.

Intestinal perforation occurs. The bowel can be grazed leading to peritonitis, abscess formation, and sepsis. Puncture of the bladder, ureters, and liver has been reported.

In summary, if an organ is in the peritoneal cavity, then it has been damaged at laparoscopy.

Anaesthetic problems associated with laparoscopy (Box 22.4)

There are several implications for the anaesthetist with laparoscopic surgery. These are listed in Box 22.4.

> ## Box 22.4 Anaesthetic problems of laparoscopic surgery
>
> - Aspiration of gastric contents
> - Position of patient
> - Nerve injury
> - Conversion to laparotomy
> - Postoperative pain relief
> - Anaesthetic technique

It is often assumed that the Trendelenberg position and a pneumoperitoneum will lead to an increased risk of passive regurgitation of gastric contents. However, the lower oesophageal sphincter pressure alters little and the risk is low but present.

The patient is often in a steep Trendelenberg position for gynaecological surgery, but may be in a head-up position for abdominal surgery. Occasionally, both are employed in the same patient.

121

Nerve damage can occur: the common peroneal nerve, femoral nerve, and the brachial plexus are at risk.

A small number of patients proceed to laparotomy. The anaesthetist should be prepared for this possibility at the start of the procedure.

Postoperative pain can be decreased by infiltrating with local anaesthetic the wounds made by the trochar. Shoulder tip pain may occur from diaphragmatic irritation by the gas.

Many anaesthetic techniques have been used for laparoscopy. Epidural and spinal anaesthesia are not well tolerated because of the discomfort from peritoneal distension and respiratory stimulation. General anaesthesia is used frequently. The safest and preferred technique is endotracheal intubation and ventilation of the patient. This allows abdominal wall relaxation and decreases the effects of diaphragmatic splinting on respiratory function. The risk of gastric aspiration is minimised and, should a laparotomy ensue, you are prepared. Emergency laparoscopic surgery necessitates a rapid sequence induction technique. Adequate venous access is essential for laparoscopic anaesthesia as profound haemorrhage can occur.

Ectopic pregnancy

Ectopic pregnancy is sometimes a life-threatening emergency. The relevant anaesthetic considerations are shown in Box 22.5.

Box 22.5   Anaesthetic considerations in ectopic pregnancy

- Patient empathy
- Emergency anaesthesia
- Haemorrhage
- Pregnancy
- Surgical technique—laparotomy or laparoscopy
- Postoperative analgesia

Patients are often very upset; be kind. There may be considerable blood loss and full resuscitation should occur before induction of anaesthesia. Adequate blood must be available, but occasionally it is necessary to start surgery without this facility to save life. Insert a wide bore intravenous cannula before induction; do not rely on a cannula placed by a gynaecologist.

A rapid sequence induction technique is used to avoid gastric aspiration. The surgical procedure may be done by a laparotomy, or by a laparoscopic technique. Appropriate postoperative analgesia should be prescribed.

Evacuation of retained products of conception (ERPC)

This operation is very common and the anaesthetic considerations are shown in Box 22.6.

> ## Box 22.6   Anaesthetic considerations for ERPC
>
> - Patient empathy
> - Timing of surgery
> - Pregnancy
> - Haemorrhage
> - Oxytocic drugs
> - Infection
> - Type of anaesthesia
>   - regional or general
>   - need for endotracheal intubation

Again a sympathetic approach to the patient is essential. An ERPC is not an emergency procedure and, in the absence of haemorrhage, should be undertaken during routine operating time. The risks of the procedure are haemorrhage, infection, and uterine perforation. Oxytocic drugs are used to contract the uterus. Syntocinon is commonly used as a bolus injection and occasionally causes hypotension. Ergometrine contracts smooth muscle and can provoke vomiting.

Regional anaesthesia can be used for ERPC (epidural, spinal) and a level of analgesia to T10 is required. Usually the surgery is carried out under general anaesthesia. There are two special considerations. The first relates to the pregnant patient and the full stomach. If the procedure is not an emergency, the patient is not suffering from any specific symptoms of pregnancy, such as heartburn, and the patient is <16 weeks pregnant, then endotracheal intubation is unnecessary. If the patient is >16 weeks pregnant, a rapid sequence induction and endotracheal intubation is recommended.

Secondly, volatile anaesthetic agents relax the uterus. This increases blood loss and the risk of perforation of the uterus. Therefore, some anaesthetists will not use volatile agents. Instead, intravenous anaesthesia (propofol) with supplementation by nitrous oxide and oxygen is given.

Laparotomy

General anaesthesia for operations on the uterus and the ovaries is similar to that described in abdominal anaesthesia (Chapter 24).

Regional anaesthesia is an excellent technique for gynaecological surgery, with the benefit of good postoperative analgesia. The innervation of the uterus is up to T10. If manipulation of the bowel occurs, or there is haemorrhage in the paracolic gutters, the patient may experience discomfort. An extension of neural blockade to T4 (as for a Caesarean section) is then needed to relieve pain.

Conclusion

You will undertake a lot of anaesthesia for gynaecological surgery in the early months of your career. Always assume that the gynaecologists have no knowledge of anything that occurs outside the pelvis, preoperative assessment must be meticulous, and do not underestimate their ability to cause severe blood loss.

23: Anaesthesia for urological surgery

Urological surgical lists provide supervised experience in anaesthetising elderly patients with medical problems. They are useful for learning basic regional techniques such as spinal anaesthesia.

Transurethral resection of the prostate (TURP)

This involves resection of the prostate by a modified cystoscope which cuts tissue and coagulates blood vessels. The procedure is facilitated by means of irrigating fluid which flows through the cystoscope. This fluid washes blood away from the cut prostatic tissue so that the operative site can be seen. Further resection occurs and any bleeding venous sinuses are coagulated. The requirements of the irrigating fluid are shown in Box 23.1.

> **Box 23.1 Requirements for urological irrigating fluid**
>
> - Prevents dispersal of electrical current
> - Clear for visibility
> - Sterile
> - Nontoxic locally
> - Nontoxic systemically
> - Isothermic
> - Isotonic
> - Non-haemolytic
> - Inexpensive

The current from the diathermy must not be spread to the bladder wall through the irrigating fluid. The fluid must be nontoxic, especially if absorbed through the open venous sinuses of the prostate. The solution used in current practice is glycine 1·5% which is slightly hypotonic (2·1% is isotonic).

Irrigation is performed under hydrostatic pressure during prostatic resection and some intravenous absorption of the glycine will take place through the prostatic, venous sinuses. The amount of irrigating fluid absorbed depends on several factors (Box 23.2).

Box 23.2   Factors influencing the absorption of glycine

- Hydrostatic pressure of the irrigating fluid
- Number and size of the venous sinuses opened
- Duration of surgery
- Venous pressure at the irrigant–blood interface

The height of the glycine should be less than 70 cm above the patient. Symptoms of glycine absorption may take as little as 15 min to appear and up to 2 l of fluid can be absorbed. Usually surgery is restricted to a duration of 1 hour only.

Anaesthetic considerations for TURP are shown in Box 23.3.

Box 23.3   Anaesthetic problems for TURP

- Elderly population
- Concurrent diseases
- Dilutional hyponatraemia and overhydration (TURP syndrome)
- Haemolysis
- Haemorrhage
- Infection
- Patient position
- Hypothermia
- Perforation of bladder
- Erection
- Adductor spasm
- Burns and explosions
- Postoperative clot retention

Elderly men often have severe medical problems which must be assessed and treated preoperatively. If prostatic obstruction is chronic, renal impairment may be present.

TURP syndrome

The absorption intravenously of the irrigating fluid, if severe, causes iatrogenic water intoxication—the TURP syndrome. This can present in a number of ways and is more easily detected in an awake patient having regional anaesthesia than in one undergoing general anaesthesia. Symptoms and signs of the TURP syndrome are shown in Box 23.4.

Box 23.4   Symptoms and signs of acute water intoxication (TURP syndrome)

- Agitation
- Restlessness
- Confusion
- Vomiting
- Blurred vision
- Transient blindness
- Coma
- Convulsions
- Unexplained bradycardia
- Unexplained hypotension
- Unexplained hypertension
- Pulmonary oedema
- ECG changes
- Asystole

Signs of cerebral irritation are usually seen first and vomiting is a consistent feature. Under general anaesthesia ECG changes, such as a wide QRS complex, T wave inversion, and rarely ventricular tachycardia and asystole, may be the only signs.

If water intoxication is suspected, the blood tests shown in Box 23.5 should be done immediately.

Box 23.5   Blood tests in suspected TURP syndrome

- Haemoglobin/haematocrit
- Serum osmolality
- Plasma sodium
- Plasma potassium
- Plasma glycine
- Plasma ammonia

The most important findings are a low plasma sodium concentration, low osmolality, and low haemoglobin concentration. A sodium concentration of <120 mmol/l is associated with significant symptoms and signs. The plasma ammonia and glycine values will not be immediately available, but will confirm the absorption of the glycine.

Treatment should be aimed at prevention and then management of the syndrome (Box 23.6). Treatment of *acute* intoxication is undertaken rapidly; the prompt reversal of *chronic* water intoxication can result in cerebral pontine myelosis.

Box 23.6   Management of water intoxication in TURP syndrome

- Prevention
  - correct intravenous fluid of choice (avoid 5% glucose, glucose/saline solutions)
  - short duration of surgery by competent surgeon

- Treatment
  - stop surgery if possible
  - oxygen
  - CVP measurement
  - diuresis
  - intravenous sodium solutions
  - circulatory support
  - symptom control

Sodium chloride solution (0·9%) or colloids such as gelofusine are the intravenous fluid of choice for TURP.

The TURP syndrome is a medical emergency and needs experienced anaesthetic help. Diuretic therapy is the mainstay of treatment and frusemide is the agent of choice; 0·9% sodium chloride or even hypertonic saline should be given judiciously to increase the plasma sodium concentration.

Other anaesthetic problems

Haemolysis presents in a similar way to a transfusion reaction. The patient may complain of weakness, rigors, and chest pain, and become hypertensive. Haemoglobinaemia, haemoglobinuria, and anaemia may occur, with acute tubular necrosis. Treatment should be directed towards obtaining a diuresis and specific correction of the haematological and biochemical abnormalities.

Haemorrhage is not uncommon and blood loss is difficult to assess since the blood is diluted with irrigating fluid. The usual methods of estimating blood loss are inappropriate. Careful assessment of the circulation by conventional means is used. If methods of estimating the haemoglobin concentration of the irrigating fluid are available, then the blood loss can be calculated.

Bacteraemia and septicaemia can result from instrumentation and there is always the risk of sudden postoperative septicaemia. Antibiotics, especially gentamicin, are given on induction to reduce this risk.

The patient is in the lithotomy position, which assists venous return. When the patient's legs are placed horizontally at the end of surgery, especially when regional techniques are used, the arterial pressure often declines as a result of the decreased venous return.

Irrigating fluids during prolonged surgery cause hypothermia. Occasionally perforation of the bladder can occur.

Erection, which usually occurs when regional anaesthesia is used, prevents instrumentation of the penis and surgery is not possible. Ketamine in small incremental doses of 5–10 mg i.v. is reputed to help with this irritating and embarrassing problem.

If the obturator nerve is stimulated accidentally by the surgeon, adductor spasm occurs. Sudden closure of the thighs commands the attention of the surgeon.

There is always a slight risk of burns and explosions since the diathermy carries high frequency current at a power of up to 400 W with a voltage of 2000 V.

If clot retention occurs postoperatively, the urinary catheter will block. The irrigating fluid must be turned off until the clot is removed by flushing the catheter and bladder. If the irrigating fluid is kept running, the bladder will fill and the irrigating fluid will be absorbed through the prostatic venous plexus. This is painful and dangerous, with the risk of TURP syndrome.

The operation is not usually painful and, after regional anaesthesia, little further pain relief is needed.

The choices of anaesthesia for TURP are shown in Box 23.7.

Box 23.7   Anaesthesia for TURP

- Regional anaesthesia ($\pm$ sedation)
  - spinal
  - epidural
  - caudal

- General anaesthesia
  - spontaneous ventilation
  - controlled ventilation

Regional anaesthesia must reach the level of T10 to prevent pain from bladder distension. General and regional anaesthesia are sometimes combined.

The advantages and disadvantages of regional anaesthesia are shown in Box 23.8.

Box 23.8 Advantages and disadvantages of regional anaesthesia for TURP

- Advantages
  - avoids complications of general anaesthesia
  - better postoperative analgesia
  - early recognition of TURP syndrome
  - less deep vein thrombosis
  - earlier mobilisation
  - less bleeding intraoperatively
  - better operating field

- Disadvantages
  - less control of arterial pressure
  - headaches
  - difficult to position elderly patient for block
  - patient preference for unconsciousness

The advantages and disadvantages of general anaesthesia are shown in Box 23.9.

Box 23.9 Advantages and disadvantages of general anaesthesia for TURP

- Advantages
  - often faster
  - patient preference
  - surgeon preference
  - better control of arterial pressure
  - avoids complications of regional anaesthesia

- Disadvantages
  - slower recovery period
  - postoperative analgesia less good
  - slower mobilisation
  - slower recognition of TURP syndrome
  - risk of general anaesthetic complications

Cystoscopic procedures

Cystoscopy can be done with flexible or rigid cystoscopes on an inpatient or outpatient list, under either general or local anaesthesia. Rigid cystoscopy is usually performed under general anaesthesia. The surgical requirement for resection, or biopsy, of the bladder wall is that the patient does not cough or strain unexpectedly, and that respiration is not forced (a smooth anaesthetic with a perfect airway). Otherwise, the bowel will move the bladder wall and there is a risk of perforation. A laparotomy will be required to repair the bladder.

Circumcision

Circumcision, whether in a child or adult, is a painful operation and good postoperative analgesia must be provided. The most common methods are either a caudal anaesthetic, which may result in leg weakness for several hours, or a penile nerve block. For the latter, local anaesthetic is injected in the midline below the symphysis pubis with the risk of intravascular injection.

Operations on testicles

Torsion of the testes is a surgical emergency and appropriate precautions must be undertaken (Chapter 21). The operation is usually conducted under general anaesthesia. If regional anaesthesia is used, neuronal blockade to the level of T9 is required.

Renal surgery

Specific problems of renal surgery are shown in Box 23.10.

Box 23.10   Specific considerations in renal surgery

- Position of patient
- Difficult access to intravenous cannulae
- Muscle relaxation
- Haemorrhage
- Pneumothorax
- Postoperative analgesia

The patient may be supine or in a lateral, jack-knife position. Good muscular relaxation is a surgical requirement. Intraoperative haemorrhage may be considerable. The risk of a pneumothorax should not be underestimated (Chapter 16). Good postoperative analgesia is essential and epidural analgesia is often used. A combination of general anaesthesia and regional anaesthesia (epidural) is particularly appropriate for renal surgery.

Conclusion

Urological surgical lists are often unpopular with trainees, but anaesthesia for these patients is challenging. Patients are usually male, elderly, with medical problems and the surgery has some specific complications. Careful preoperative assessment is essential and regional anaesthesia is often appropriate.

One author spent many happy years helping relieve obstruction in old men.

24: Anaesthesia for abdominal surgery

General considerations

Laparoscopic techniques are increasingly common in abdominal surgery, for example laparoscopic cholecystectomy and laparoscopically-assisted colectomy. The anaesthetic implications of laparoscopic surgery are discussed in Chapter 22. Careful anaesthetic management of the patient is essential in abdominal surgery, as major errors result in increased patient morbidity and even mortality.

In addition to routine preoperative assessment, particular attention should be given to the problems listed in Box 24.1.

> **Box 24.1 Specific preoperative problems in abdominal surgery**
>
> - Fluid balance
> - Electrolyte disorders
> - Full stomach
> - Accompanying disease(s)
> - Airway assessment
> - Drugs

Fluid balance is often difficult to assess. A patient presenting with emergency bowel obstruction may have up to 2–3 l of fluid sequestered in the bowel. Even in elective bowel surgery, the bowel is prepared by the liberal use of enemas before surgery. These patients are invariably dehydrated unless care is taken to provide adequate preoperative intravenous hydration.

Vomiting can lead to dehydration and is one of the many causes of electrolyte disturbances in these patients. Hypokalaemia must be corrected before surgery, to avoid the complications listed in Box 24.2.

A thorough assessment of the airway is mandatory and patients at risk of regurgitation or aspiration should have a rapid sequence induction.

Some diseases of the gut, such as ulcerative colitis and Crohn's disease, are multisystem diseases in which the skin, joints, eyes, mouth, and renal

> **Box 24.2   Complications of hypokalaemia**
>
> - Arrhythmias
> - Potentiation of competitive neuromuscular blocking drugs
> - Prolonged ileus
> - Respiratory muscle weakness
> - Decreased inotropsim

systems may be affected. These patients are often receiving steroid therapy and appropriate steroid cover must be provided in the perioperative period. For most patients hydrocortisone 25 mg i.v. at induction followed by 100 mg i.v./24 hours until oral therapy is restarted is sufficient. Occasionally it is necessary to give more hydrocortisone to maintain immune suppression during an acute illness. For example, a patient receiving 60 mg prednisolone/day should receive an equivalent dose of hydrocortisone (60 mg × 4 = 240 mg).

The perioperative problems of abdominal surgery are shown on Box 24.3.

> **Box 24.3   Perioperative considerations for abdominal surgery**
>
> - Rapid sequence induction of anaesthesia
> - Venous access
> - Muscular relaxation
> - Vagal responses to surgery
> - Infection
> - Position of the patient
> - Drugs
> - Body temperature
> - Adjunct regional analgesia
> - Haemorrhage + fluid therapy

Most abdominal surgery requires adequate muscular relaxation. Sudden traction of viscera can stimulate vagally mediated reflexes and result in a bradycardia. Bowel inflammation, perforation, and obstruction can lead to septicaemia, and antibiotics such as gentamicin, cefuroxime, and metronidazole are often given pre- and intraoperatively. Gentamicin, an aminoglycoside antibiotic, theoretically potentiates the action of competitive neuromuscular blocking drugs. It is obviously a rare occurrence as neither author has encountered this problem.

Patients in the Lloyd Davies position can suffer nerve damage to the legs and these should be padded appropriately. The common peroneal nerve at the top of the fibula is particularly at risk and foot drop may occur postoperatively. Access to the airway and the venous cannula is often difficult.

Certain drugs affect bowel motility. Opioids increase circular smooth muscle contractility of the gut and hence bowel tone, decreasing propulsive activity. Nitrous oxide distends gas-filled cavities such as the bowel. Neostigmine increases gastrointestinal motility, which may threaten an intestinal anastomosis. There is little evidence, however, that the routine use of neostigmine increases the rate of anastomotic leaks after major abdominal surgery.

Heat conservation in abdominal surgical patients is important. The exposure of the viscera to air at room temperature exacerbates heat lost by radiation and convection. Temperature losses >0·5°C/h have been found, particularly when peritoneal lavage is used. Heat loss should be prevented with hot air warming blankets, heat and moisture filters in the circuit, and the use of warming devices for intravenous fluids.

Regional anaesthetic techniques, such as epidural analgesia, are often used to provide intraoperative and postoperative analgesia. Major bowel surgery cannot be carried out with these techniques alone unless a block above T4 is achieved. Regional anaesthesia is commonly used to supplement general anaesthesia with controlled ventilation for major surgery. The integrity of the bowel anastomosis is critically important in abdominal surgery. An adequate circulating blood volume and arterial pressure must be maintained to ensure that blood flow to the gut is not compromised.

Particular postoperative problems are shown in Box 24.4.

Box 24.4   Specific postoperative problems in abdominal surgery

- Analgesia
- Fluid balance
- Oxygen therapy
- High-dependency nursing care

Pain after laparotomy can result in hypoventilation, lung collapse, and infection. Good postoperative analgesia is important and regional anaesthesia is often used. Patient controlled analgesia and subcutaneous opiate infusions are alternative techniques.

Careful fluid balance is important as an ileus postoperatively can cause large fluid losses to be missed. Meticulous attention to urine output (>0·5 ml/kg/h) and central venous and arterial pressure measurement will detect postoperative dehydration.

Intrapulmonary shunts and hypoventilation after abdominal surgery are common and may persist for up to 72 h after surgery. Postoperative oxygen therapy may be needed during this time.

Appropriate nursing care must be provided after major abdominal surgery. This usually necessitates admission to a high dependency unit or intensive therapy unit.

Anal surgery

Operations in the anal region, such as anal stretch, drainage of perianal abscess, excision of pilonidal sinus, haemorrhoidectomy, and lateral sphincterotomy can cause anaesthetic difficulties.

The surgeon often asks that the anal sphincter tone is not altered and this precludes techniques using muscle relaxants and epidural, spinal, and caudal anaesthesia, as they all relax the anal sphincter. The operations are short in duration but very painful. Profound anaesthesia is necessary, but the patient must awaken rapidly after surgery and be pain free. A regional technique applied at the end of surgery, such as local anaesthetic infiltration or caudal anaesthesia, is helpful.

The anaesthetic problems of anal surgery are shown in Box 24.5.

> **Box 24.5 Anaesthetic problems of anal surgery**
> - Normal anal sphincter tone
> - Depth of anaesthesia
> - Intraoperative analgesia
> - Position of patient
> - Arrhythmias
> - Laryngospasm
> - Postoperative analgesia

The patient is usually placed in the lithotomy position; access to the venous cannula and airway may be difficult. If the depth of general anaesthesia is inadequate, arrhythmias, especially bradycardia, and laryngospasm may occur with the application of a painful stimulus. The anaesthetic requires, therefore, skill and simplicity. Opiate premedication is often used, and anaesthesia conducted with a suitable induction agent, opiate, and nitrous oxide, oxygen, and a volatile agent. Atropine and suxamethonium *must* be available.

It is embarrassing for a previously smooth anaesthetic to degenerate into a noisy shambles as the patient develops laryngospasm when the haemorrhoid is clamped firmly by the surgeon. The management of laryngospasm is discussed in Chapter 17.

Conclusion

Major abdominal surgery is difficult. The patients are often ill, with pre-existing fluid and electrolyte problems. Careful preoperative assessment and resuscitation, and high quality postoperative care are essential. A combination of general and regional anaesthesia is often appropriate. Beware anal surgery—a small orifice that causes big problems (anaesthetically, of course).

25: Anaesthesia for dental and ENT surgery

The problems of anaesthetising for surgical procedures in and near the airway are common to both dental and ENT surgery.

Shared airway

A patent, secure airway is essential for safe anaesthetic practice. If possible, the tracheal tube or laryngeal mask airway should not protrude into the surgical field. Access to the airway is lost once the patient is draped and surgery started. The anaesthetic circuit is often long (and occasionally bulky) as the anaesthetic machine is placed at the feet of the patient. Two major problems may arise:

- the weight of the circuit can pull out or kink the endotracheal tube: care must be taken to ensure that the circuit is supported to avoid drag;
- the surgeon may obstruct the tracheal tube when operating.

If the airway is lost, surgery must be stopped and appropriate adjustments made. Most surgeons understand the problems of the shared airway and are cooperative. However, one author had the alarming experience of the surgeon suddenly handing him the endotracheal tube because it was interfering with the surgery.

Venous access is also restricted and extension tubing on an intravenous cannula is essential.

Dental anaesthesia

Anaesthesia in the dental chair had a justifiable reputation as one of the major sporting events in anaesthetic practice. At present, dental anaesthesia is conducted either in hospital, or in fully equipped premises, usually as day-stay surgery. The problems of dental anaesthesia are the same, irrespective of the place and duration of surgery. Dental operations can take only a few seconds, but you must provide suitable anaesthesia in an appropriate, safe environment.

There are many possible anaesthetic techniques for dental surgery (Box 25.1).

> **Box 25.1   Anaesthetic techniques for dental surgery**
>
> - Local anaesthesia
> - Local anaesthesia and sedation
> - Sedation
>   - intravenous
>   - inhalational
> - General anaesthesia
> - General anaesthesia and local anaesthesia

The teeth are supplied by branches of the trigeminal nerve and dental surgeons are adroit at blocking the superior and inferior alveolar nerves at specific sites. Dental surgeons use prilocaine with adrenaline or felypressin (a less toxic vasoconstrictor than adrenaline). If sedation is used, the patient must be able to talk to the anaesthetist or dental surgeon. Intravenous benzodiazepines are used frequently to provide sedation; occasionally Entonox (50% N_2O:50% O_2) is inhaled.

There are many important considerations for general anaesthesia in dental surgery (Box 25.2).

> **Box 25.2   Considerations for general anaesthesia in dental surgery**
>
> - Antisialogue
> - Method of induction
> - Type of tracheal tube
> - Throat packs
> - Surgical infiltration of local anaesthetic with felypressin
> - Patient position—usually supine
> - Mouth props
> - Maintenance of anaesthesia
> - Haemorrhage
> - Arrhythmias
> - Postoperative analgesia
> - Laryngospasm
> - Antibiotics
> - Decrease in local swelling with steroids

Surgeons prefer a dry mouth, as it makes surgery easier. An anticholinergic drug in the premedication also protects against a bradycardia that often occurs during surgery. An intravenous induction is used if there are no difficulties with the airway. Control of the airway is obtained with a nasotracheal tube, and throat packs are inserted before surgery to collect blood and debris. It is easy to inadvertently leave the throat packs in at the end of surgery—obstruction of the airway occurs. One author always ties one end of the pack to the nasotracheal tube, or circuit, to act as an obvious reminder.

Complications during and after dental surgery are common. Severe haemorrhage is fortunately rare after dental surgery, but if there is any doubt about the adequacy of haemostasis then the patient must be kept in hospital under close observation. Arrhythmias are common (30% of patients) and can continue in the postoperative period. Oedema can be minimised by the use of steroids before surgery. Extubation of the trachea can be undertaken under light or deep anaesthesia. Under deep anaesthesia the patient is less likely to develop laryngospasm, but is more likely to aspirate vomit, blood, or debris. Under light anaesthesia the patient has adequate protective reflexes, but is more prone to laryngospasm. We prefer the latter technique.

Emergency dental anaesthesia

Emergency dental anaesthesia should not be underestimated; get help from senior anaesthetists. The principal problem in patients with a dental abscess or mandibular fractures is difficulty in opening the mouth and hence the difficulty with intubation. Fibreoptic laryngoscopy and intubation, or an inhalational induction followed by blind nasal intubation, is often necessary in these patients. Muscle relaxants must not be given until patency and control of the airway is secured.

Vigorous antibiotic therapy may decrease the infection and the urgency of the surgery should be discussed with the dental surgeon. Only rarely is it a life-threatening emergency. If the airway is not safe postoperatively, the patient should be managed in an Intensive Therapy or High Dependency Unit.

> **Box 25.3   Anaesthetic considerations for tonsillectomy**
>
> - Child—problems with parents
> - Premedication
> - Induction of anaesthesia
> - Type of tracheal tube
> - Use of Boyle Davis gag
> - Postoperative analgesia
> - Laryngospasm
> - Postoperative haemorrhage

ENT anaesthesia

The trainee is frequently introduced to anaesthesia for children on ENT lists. The anaesthetic problems of a child undergoing tonsillectomy and adenoidectomy are shown in Box 25.3.

A child with anxious parents needs special support. The parents are often present in the anaesthetic room during the induction of anaesthesia, which is undertaken either by the inhalational or intravenous route. Sedative premedication is helpful. Oral trimeprazine syrup, oral atropine and topical EMLA cream are used commonly. A preformed endotracheal tube (commonly a RAE tube) minimises, but does not exclude the risk of the Boyle Davis gag kinking and obstructing the tube. Analgesia is given intravenously during surgery to decrease pain on emergence from anaesthesia. As in dental surgery, extubation can be carried out with the patient lightly or deeply anaesthetised. Laryngospasm is again a hazard. Postoperative haemorrhage is always a potential problem (see below).

The bleeding tonsil

Haemorrhage after a tonsillectomy is a serious complication and senior assistance must be sought. The anaesthetic problems are summarised in Box 25.4.

> **Box 25.4 Anaesthetic problems in the bleeding tonsil**
>
> - Senior help essential
> - Occult haemorrhage
> - Full stomach
> - Patient often hypovolaemic
> - Resuscitation
> - Repeated anaesthesia
> - Method of induction
>   - inhalation
>   - intravenous
> - Secure airway
> - Postoperative care

There may not be much visible evidence of haemorrhage; often all the blood is swallowed. If this occurs the stomach can contain a large amount of coagulated blood. A nasogastric tube will not remove this blood and aggravates the traumatised pharynx; it should not be used. The patient may be hypovolaemic, and full, appropriate resuscitation must occur before surgery.

There is debate about the method of facilitating tracheal intubation. An inhalational induction, with the patient head down in the left lateral

141

position, maintains control of the airway at all times and any bleeding trickles out of the mouth under gravity. A rapid sequence induction may be unsafe if there is blood, or a haematoma, in the pharynx, since the airway may become obstructed before the trachea is intubated. Although we prefer the former method, we have not seen serious sequelae from a rapid sequence induction.

A patient who has received two anaesthetics in a short time and required resuscitation should be managed in a High Dependency Unit or even Intensive Therapy Unit postoperatively.

Ear surgery

Minor endoscopic procedures on the ear are conducted with the patient breathing spontaneously through a well secured and correctly positioned laryngeal mask. More complex middle ear or mastoid operations have special problems (Box 25.5).

Box 25.5 Anaesthetic considerations for middle ear surgery

- Sedative premedication
- Avoidance of preoperative tachycardia
- Shared airway
- Prolonged surgery
- Use of nitrous oxide
- Hypotensive anaesthesia
- Postoperative vomiting
- Postoperative analgesia

The patient should arrive in the anaesthetic room sedated and with a normal heart rate. The avoidance of a tachycardia makes hypotensive anaesthesia easier to achieve. Nitrous oxide diffuses into air-filled spaces and in some surgical procedures causes difficulties. Many anaesthetists avoid nitrous oxide for middle ear surgery. Postoperative vomiting can be severe and potent antiemetics are essential.

Induced hypotension is often used in these patients to decrease haemorrhage and improve the surgical field under the operating microscope. It is only suitable for patients without major cardiovascular disease and mean arterial pressures less than 60 mm Hg are unnecessary. The techniques available are shown in Box 25.6.

Box 25.6   Techniques for induced hypotension

- No obstruction to venous outflow
- No coughing or straining (increases venous pressure)
- Head-up tilt
- Use of intermittent positive pressure ventilation
- Intra-arterial monitoring essential
- Specific hypotensive drugs
  - labetalol
  - nitroprusside
  - nitroglycerine

Conclusion

Sharing the airway with the surgeon is exciting; it ensures the vigilance of the anaesthetist. It is very difficult for a dental or ENT surgeon to kill the patient, other than by obstructing or dislodging the tracheal tube. If control and patency of the airway is lost, move the surgeon *immediately* and sort out the problem.

26: Anaesthesia for orthopaedic surgery

In the bad old days a trainee anaesthetist spent long hours in the evening and night watching young orthopaedic surgeons struggle with "emergency" cases. Fortunately it has been agreed that patients with, for example, hip fractures need their surgery performed as soon as practically possible, but in the safest environment. The National Confidential Enquiry into Perioperative Deaths (NCEPOD) recommends that such surgery should not be carried out by inexperienced surgeons and anaesthetists in the night. This work should be done on designated trauma lists during the day by appropriately trained staff.

General considerations

The general considerations of anaesthesia for orthopaedic surgery are shown in Box 26.1.

Box 26.1   General considerations in orthopaedic anaesthesia

- Age
- Trauma or elective
- Concomitant injury or disease
- Use of tourniquet
- Infection
- Haemorrhage
- Methylmethacrylate cement
- Deep vein thrombosis prophylaxis
- Fat embolism

The extremes of the age range appear for orthopaedic surgery. Young people present commonly with trauma, whilst elderly patients often present for joint arthroplasty or with a fractured femoral neck. Age is not a contraindication to surgery and you should learn to assess patients in terms of their *biological* age and not *chronological* age. Providing there are no major medical problems, elderly patients with hip fractures should have surgery on the earliest available trauma list. Otherwise, bed rest is associated with weakness, confusion, chest infection, and deep vein thrombosis, and recovery from the delayed surgery is prolonged. Postoperative mortality and morbidity remain high in these patients.

After major trauma, emergency surgery on patients with compound fractures is common. Associated spinal and neck injuries must be sought and appropriate treatment instituted before induction of anaesthesia. Traumatic injuries, such as fractured ribs and a fractured pelvis, are often associated with damage to abdominal viscera such as the spleen and liver.

Orthopaedic surgery in the elderly is usually complicated by concomitant diseases. Patients for joint arthroplasties may have medical problems such as rheumatoid arthritis. Patients with hip fractures may simply have tripped and fallen, but the fall may have followed a cerebral ischaemic attack or a cardiac arrhythmia. Even carpal tunnel syndrome is sometimes associated with hypothyroidism, acromegaly, and pregnancy.

Tourniquets are used commonly to exsanguinate the limb and keep blood out of the operative field. They must be placed carefully to avoid creasing of the skin which results in irritation and blister formation. Tourniquets are not used in people with sickle cell disease, for fear of provoking a sickle crisis. The recommended maximum duration of tourniquet time is 90 min. Pressures used are 33–40 kPa (250–300 mm Hg) for the arm and 46–53 kPa (350–400 mm Hg) for the leg. They must be fixed securely to prevent loosening. Haemorrhage after release of the tourniquet can be brisk. Red cell transfusion is usual after major traumatic fractures, but is now less common during and after joint arthroplasties.

The cement used in orthopaedic surgery is methylmethacrylate. This liquid monomer becomes a solid polymer after reconstitution, and heat is generated. The bone cavity should be vented as the cement is inserted to prevent embolism of bone marrow and debris. Occasionally severe hypotension occurs as the cement is inserted, although the precise mechanism is unknown. Extra vigilance is required at this time; the hypotension usually responds to the rapid administration of intravenous fluid. Occasionally vasopressors are required.

Deep vein thrombosis remains the cause of significant morbidity and mortality after orthopaedic surgery. Heparin prophylaxis is essential for major lower limb surgery.

Fat embolism occurs occasionally after trauma or surgery involving the pelvis or long bones (0·5–2% patients). The initial symptoms and signs are as those of pulmonary thromboembolism. Fatty acid release causes diminished mental status, hypoxaemia, petechial haemorrhages, and disseminated intravascular coagulation.

145

Anaesthesia for specific operations

Arm surgery

Arm surgery can be carried out under regional anaesthesia, general anaesthesia, or a combination of both. The indications and contraindications of each technique need to be considered, together with the wishes of the patient and the surgeon. Anaesthetic considerations and techniques are shown in Box 26.2.

Box 26.2   Anaesthetic considerations and techniques for arm surgery

- Intravenous access
- Use of tourniquet
- Duration of surgery
- Concomitant diseases
- Patient preference
- Surgeon preference
- Emergency or elective
- Regional anaesthesia ± sedation
  - brachial plexus block
  - individual nerve blocks at elbow
  - intravenous regional anaesthesia
  - local anaesthetic injection at operative site
- General anaesthesia
  - ? endotracheal intubation
  - spontaneous ventilation or controlled ventilation

Regional anaesthesia avoids the drowsiness, nausea, and vomiting of general anaesthesia, but can be difficult to perform, is slow in onset, and occasionally results in major complications such as pneumothorax and inadvertent intravascular injection (brachial plexus block). Nevertheless, if the patient and surgeon agree, we prefer regional rather than general anaesthesia.

Leg surgery

The anaesthetic considerations and techniques available for hip surgery are shown in Box 26.3.

Elderly patients have fragile skin which must be cared for appropriately. Nerve palsies can arise and care must be taken to avoid damage to the ulnar nerves; suitable padding should be used.

146

Box 26.3   Anaesthetic considerations and techniques for hip surgery

- Age
- Elective or emergency surgery
- Concomitant diseases
- Patient position
- Skin care
- Nerve damage from positioning of patient
- Haemorrhage
- Infection
- Methylmethacrylate cement
- General anaesthesia
  - spontaneous ventilation or controlled ventilation
- Regional anaesthesia ± sedation
  - spinal
  - epidural
  - psoas block
- Combination of general and regional anaesthesia
- Postoperative analgesia

The advantages and disadvantages of regional anaesthesia are shown in Box 26.4.

Box 26.4   Advantages and disadvantages of regional anaesthesia for hip surgery

- Advantages
  - no risks from general anaesthesia
  - decreased blood loss
  - decreased risk of deep vein thrombosis
  - better immediate postoperative analgesia
  - earlier mobilisation
  - decreased risk of respiratory infection
  - less vomiting and mental confusion

- Disadvantages
  - surgeon preference
  - patient preference
  - complications of technique used
    - hypotension
    - headache
    - difficult to perform in elderly

The advantages and disadvantages of general anaesthesia for hip surgery are shown in Box 26.5.

147

Box 26.5   Advantages and disadvantages of general anaesthesia for hip surgery

- Advantages
  - often faster induction
  - patient preference
  - surgeon preference
  - better control of cardiovascular system
  - control of airway
  - avoids complications of regional anaesthesia

- Disadvantages
  - risks of general anaesthesia
  - slower recovery
  - slower mobilisation
  - more vomiting and confusion
  - increased risk of respiratory infection

We prefer regional anaesthesia, often combined with general anaesthesia, because of the proven decrease in blood loss and decreased incidence of deep vein thrombosis.

Spinal surgery

Special considerations apply to anaesthesia for spinal surgery (Box 26.6).

Box 26.6   Anaesthetic considerations for spinal surgery

- Prone position
- Care of eyes
- Type of endotracheal tube
- Difficult airway access—secure tube
- Difficult intravenous access
- Correct position of abdomen
- Specific nerve damage
- Infection
- Postoperative analgesia

Patients are usually in the prone position, and corneal abrasions and pressure on the eyes must be prevented. The endotracheal tubes used are nylon reinforced to allow bending without kinking. They often need an introducer for insertion and, as they cannot be cut to a suitable size, may inadvertently pass into the right main bronchus. The endotracheal tube must be well secured as dislodgement when the patient is prone can be disastrous. The patient must be positioned correctly, often with the use of a Montreal mattress to support the chest and prevent compression of the abdomen. Abdominal compression decreases blood flow in the vena cava, but increases flow through the epidural veins making surgery more difficult and increasing blood loss. Nerves liable to damage include the brachial plexus, ulnar nerves, nerves at the wrist, and the femoral nerves. These must be padded appropriately. These operations are often painful and appropriate postoperative analgesia must be given and discussed preoperatively with the patient. Regional anaesthesia is particularly effective.

Conclusion

Trauma and degenerative arthritic disease will ensure that orthopaedic surgery is not going to disappear. Much orthopaedic anaesthesia can be conducted with regional techniques; it is an excellent environment in which to learn these skills. Remember that orthopaedic surgeons are usually "Black and Decker" men and sometimes have only a passing acquaintance with medicine.

27: Management of the patient in the recovery area

At the end of surgery, the patient is transferred to the recovery area and is looked after by trained staff. The anaesthetist must explain what specific care is required in addition to the routine observations. The patient remains the responsibility of the anaesthetist during this time and an anaesthetist must be available immediately should any problems arise. If you have any doubts about leaving the patient in the care of the recovery staff, then you must remain with the patient. Your duty lies with the patient you have just anaesthetised—the remaining cases have to wait.

The equipment and monitoring facilities in the recovery room should be the same as in a fully equipped operating theatre.

The objectives of care in the recovery room are shown in Box 27.1.

Box 27.1   Main objectives of care in the recovery area

- Assessment of conscious level
- Management of the airway
- Pain control
- Essential monitoring and observation
- Avoidance of nausea and vomiting
- Management of shivering
- Temperature control
- Care of intravenous infusion
- Observation of surgical wound drainage
- Observation of urine output
- Oxygen therapy

Most units have guidelines on routine monitoring in the recovery area and you must be familiar with them. One member of staff per patient is mandatory in the early postoperative period. Essential monitoring consists of careful, clinical observation, and regular measurement of heart rate, arterial pressure, respiration, and oxygen saturation. These measurements may be taken as frequently as every 5 min after major surgery, but at intervals of 15 min following routine, minor surgery. In most units "routine postoperative care" means recording the vital signs every 15 min. It may be desirable to monitor the patient by means of invasive techniques, such as arterial and central venous cannulation, and suitable equipment should be available in the recovery area.

Oxygen therapy

Oxygen therapy is often given routinely in the postoperative period as hypoxaemia is an inevitable consequence of major surgery. The main causes of early postoperative hypoxaemia are shown in Box 27.2. However, hypoxaemia can persist for several days.

Box 27.2 Causes of early postoperative hypoxaemia

- Hypoventilation
  - airway obstruction
  - central respiratory depression
  - respiratory muscle weakness
- Ventilation/perfusion abnormalities
- Increased oxygen consumption
  - shivering
- Impaired response to hypoxaemia
- Decreased oxygen content
  - low cardiac output
  - low haemoglobin values

Diffusion hypoxia is a transient phenomenon that occurs at the end of anaesthesia when nitrous oxide is replaced by air. Nitrous oxide enters the alveoli from the blood very rapidly. Because nitrogen is much less soluble than nitrous oxide, expired volume exceeds inspired volume, and there is a dilutional effect on oxygen in the alveoli.

The main causes of early postoperative hypoxaemia are a degree of airway obstruction, central respiratory depression usually caused by opiates, and respiratory muscle weakness resulting from inadequate reversal of neuromuscular blocking drugs. Ventilation/perfusion abnormalities can arise after prolonged general anaesthesia and are exacerbated by factors such as obesity and pulmonary disease. Even very low concentrations of volatile anaesthetic agents impair the ventilatory response to hypoxaemia.

Oxygen is administered usually by a mask; either a fixed performance or variable performance device.

Fixed performance oxygen masks

These masks provide an accurate inspired oxygen concentration which is independent of the patient's ventilation because the flow rate of fresh gas delivered is higher than the patient's inspiratory flow rate. They work on the principle of high air flow oxygen enrichment (HAFOE). Air is entrained in oxygen by means of the Venturi principle to provide accurate concentrations of 24, 28, 35, 40, and 60% oxygen, depending on which mask is used. The flow rates of oxygen required for these concentrations are written on the side of each mask. Such masks, for example, the Ventimask, are expensive and are indicated when a precise concentration of oxygen needs to be given, such as in chronic obstructive lung disease. Following routine anaesthesia cheaper masks are used which are of variable performance.

Variable performance oxygen masks

Variable performance masks, such as the Hudson mask, are dependent on the patient's inspiratory flow rate, the oxygen flow rate, and the duration of the expiratory pause. Nasal cannulae function in a similar way. If a patient is breathing normally then an oxygen flow of 4 l/min will provide an inspired oxygen concentration of about 40%. If necessary, this can be checked with an oxygen analyser.

If an inspired oxygen concentration >60% is required, it cannot usually be given by a disposable oxygen mask. An anaesthetic face mask is necessary.

Criteria for discharge from the recovery room are becoming common. The main points of anaesthetic relevance are shown in Box 27.3.

Box 27.3   Typical criteria for discharge from recovery

- Patient awake and responds appropriately to commands
- Upper airway patent and reflexes present
- Respiration satisfactory
- Cardiovascular stability
- Pain control adequate, not vomiting

Conclusion

The care of the patient in the recovery room remains the responsibility of the anaesthetist, who must be available to deal with any complications that may arise. The anaesthetist is also responsible for the discharge of the patient from the recovery area to the ward and increasingly this is a formal, documented procedure.

28: Postoperative analgesia

Pain is a subjective response to noxious stimuli and patients vary greatly in their need for analgesia after surgery. For example, the amount of morphine requested postoperatively has been found to vary ten-fold after the same operation. Analgesic regimens must take into account this unpredictable response. Acute pain teams are a popular, recent development in anaesthetic practice and have drawn attention to past failings in the provision of adequate, postoperative analgesia.

The advantages claimed for good analgesia are shown in Box 28.1.

Box 28.1   Claimed advantages of good postoperative analgesia

- Humanitarian reasons
- Psychological reasons
- Less respiratory complications
- Less adverse cardiovascular responses
- Less autonomic complications (sweating, vomiting)
- Earlier mobilisation
- Less deep vein thrombosis
- Earlier return to normal life style/work

The humanitarian and psychological advantages of good analgesia are obvious. Pain, especially after abdominal surgery, can lead to deterioration in respiratory function from a reduction in ventilatory capacity and an inability to cough. Pulmonary atelectasis and infection are more likely. Pain causes tachycardia and hypertension, and this may exacerbate any

153

existing myocardial ischaemia. Sweating and vomiting may accompany pain and good analgesia makes early mobilisation and rehabilitation easier.

Influences on postoperative pain

Postoperative pain is affected by many factors including those listed in Box 28.2.

Box 28.2   Factors influencing postoperative pain

- Age
- Sex
- Social class
- Anxiety
- Understanding of surgery
- Attitudes of staff
- Pain relief in other patients
- Type of surgery
- Type of anaesthesia

The elderly tolerate pain better than younger adults and women are more stoical than men. People in social classes III, IV and V tolerate pain better than those in social classes I and II. Patients with a high, preoperative, neuroticism score experience more pain. A reduction in anxiety, and education of the patient about the surgery, have been shown to decrease postoperative pain.

The attitudes of staff and the adequacy of analgesia provided for other patients on the ward are also important. Staff who are reluctant, or have little time to provide good postoperative analgesia, adversely affect the patient's recovery. Fear of the side effects of drugs (for example, addiction to opiates) is a totally unacceptable reason for the nursing staff not providing as much analgesic as required.

Methods of postoperative analgesia

An approach to the postoperative analgesic requirements of the patient must be considered during the preoperative visit. A typical plan is shown in Box 28.3.

Box 28.3   General plan of postoperative analgesia

- Preoperative assessment and discussion with patient
- Premedication
- Systemic drugs
  - nonsteroidal anti-inflammatory drugs
  - opiates
  - route
    - oral
    - intramuscular
    - intravenous
    - subcutaneous
    - rectal
  - mode of administration
    - patient-controlled or by medical staff
    - continuous versus intermittent methods
- Regional anaesthetic techniques
  - local anaesthetic agent
  - addition of opiate
  - route
    - epidural
    - spinal
    - caudal
    - specific nerve blocks
    - wound infiltration
  - mode of administration
    - single bolus at surgery/intermittent/infusion
- Miscellaneous techniques
  - steroids
  - Entonox
  - transcutaneous nerve stimulation
  - acupuncture
- Benefits versus side effects
- Follow-up

The importance of the preoperative visit and explanation to the patient of the procedures cannot be overemphasised. Consent for unusual routes of drug administration (for example, rectal in British patients) must be obtained. In some patients postoperative analgesia starts with premedication and the administration of opiates.

Systemic drugs

Nonsteroidal anti-inflammatory drugs (NSAIDs) such as aspirin, paracetamol, diclofenac, and piroxicam can be given as oral analgesics. These agents are often mixed with codeine and dihydrocodeine, which are occasionally given by themselves. The choice of drugs depends on the

155

personal preference of the anaesthetist. NSAIDs have important side effects (Box 28.4).

Box 28.4 Main side effects of NSAIDs

- Gastric ulceration
- Decreased platelet aggregation
- Drug interactions (for example, diuretics and serum potassium)
- Hypersensitivity
- Renal impairment

Morphine is the "gold standard" opiate drug and is widely used for postoperative analgesia. Pethidine is claimed to be less sedative and have relaxant properties on smooth muscle. We consider pethidine to be a potent emetic and weak analgesic and never use it. All opiates cause side effects (Box 28.5).

Box 28.5 Major side effects of systemic opiates

- Nausea and vomiting
- Sedation
- Dysphoria
- Euphoria
- Constipation
- Delayed stomach emptying
- Hallucinations

The traditional method of providing postoperative analgesia, by giving intramuscular morphine on request by the patient, has many drawbacks including intermittent analgesia and inadequate dosage. New advances in opiate administration have occurred recently.

Patient-controlled analgesia (PCA)

Syringe pumps have been devised so that the patients (not visitors, or members of staff) can administer their own analgesia intravenously. The pumps must be safe and programmed to provide sufficient analgesia after major surgery (Box 28.6). Once programmed they must be locked so that neither the syringe of opiate nor the controls are accessible. Patient controlled analgesia does not mean patient-programmed analgesia. Careful explanation to the patient about PCA is essential for the success of the technique.

> **Box 28.6   Typical regimen for intravenous morphine PCA pump**
>
> | Drug details | Regimen |
> | --- | --- |
> | Dose | 50 mg in 50 ml sodium chloride |
> | Concentration | 1 mg/ml |
> | Bolus dose | 1 mg |
> | Lock out time | 5 min |
> | Hourly dose limit | 12 mg |

In theory, if patients become too drowsy they will not push the button and so will not receive excessive doses of opiate. Despite this, staff must monitor at least hourly, the severity of the pain, the amount of analgesia used, the degree of sedation, and the respiratory rate. If the respiratory rate is <10 breaths/min or the patient too drowsy, the infusion must be stopped. The opiate antagonist, naloxone must be available and may be given in cases of severe respiratory depression, but it should be remembered that analgesia will also be reversed.

Subcutaneous infusions

· Opiates can be administered subcutaneously by continuous infusion pumps that are altered by the staff, not the patient. Morphine is given at a concentration of 2·5 mg/ml (50 mg in 20 ml sodium chloride solution). For example, the infusion is given at a rate of 1·25–3·75 mg/h. Increments of 2·5 mg can be given for breakthrough pain. Monitoring must be undertaken as described above; overdose again causes severe drowsiness and respiratory depression.

Regional techniques

Local anaesthetic drugs can be administered either as a single bolus, intermittent injections, or a continuous infusion. They can be given into the subcutaneous tissue around a wound, into joints, the pleural cavity, and in the region of the spinal cord (epidural, spinal, caudal). Opiates are often given by the epidural route, either in combination with local anaesthetics, or individually, to provide analgesia. Local anesthetics have toxic side effects and are discussed with the more common nerve blocks in Chapter 20. The balance of possible complications versus benefits must be considered.

Miscellaneous

Entonox (50% N_2O:50% O_2) is used to help alleviate the pain of short-lived procedures such as the removal of chest drains. Steroids can reduce swelling and consequently pain in dental procedures.

Transcutaneous nerve stimulators and acupuncture are used occasionally as adjuncts to other analgesic techniques.

Conclusion

Many techniques are currently available to provide pain relief after surgery. Side effects are inevitable and some of these, such as vomiting with opiates, can be distressing. It is essential that you see the effectiveness, or otherwise, of the chosen postoperative analgesic regimen and ask the patients for their opinions.

29: Management of head injuries

Patients with head injuries suffer primary brain damage at the time of the trauma. Secondary brain damage occurs after the initial insult and is caused by a decrease in cerebral perfusion and oxygenation. The anaesthetist can reduce morbidity and mortality from secondary brain damage by preventing or treating the causes listed in Box 29.1.

Box 29.1 Causes of secondary brain damage after trauma

- Hypoxaemia
- Hypercapnia
- Hypotension
- Increased cerebral venous pressure
  - coughing
  - straining
- Infection

General considerations

A rapid assessment of the patient must take place before resuscitation and treatment. Physical examination must include a careful assessment of the cervical spine as there is a high correlation between skull fractures and neck fractures. The neck should be immobilised by in-line cervical traction, or a stiff neck collar, until radiographic exclusion of a fracture has been undertaken. Life-threatening chest and abdominal injuries should be looked for carefully, and control and treatment of these should take priority over transfer, or neurosurgical intervention. Neurosurgical units are often isolated hospitals and have to transfer patients to nearby hospitals for major thoracic and abdominal surgery before neurosurgical intervention.

The airway must be cleared of blood, loose teeth, and debris and protected by tracheal intubation if necessary. Assessment of the airway is mandatory and you should assume that the patient has a full stomach. If intubation is deemed necessary, and airway assessment shows that this is likely to be successful, then a rapid sequence induction technique can be undertaken. Thiopentone and propofol attenuate the rise in intracranial pressure that occurs with laryngoscopy. Suxamethonium increases intracranial pressure transiently, but this is acceptable compared with the risks of an obstructed airway. Furthermore, hyperventilation after intubation rapidly decreases intracranial pressure. A nasogastric tube empties the stomach and should be inserted after endotracheal intubation. The reasons for endotracheal intubation in a patient with a head injury are shown in Box 29.2.

Box 29.2   Indications for endotracheal intubation in the head-injured patient

- Airway protection
  - loss of laryngeal reflexes
  - unconscious patient (GCS <8)
  - compromised airway (for example, facial injuries)
- Hypoventilation
  - hypoxaemia
  - hypercapnia
  - associated chest injury
  - associated drugs
  - airway obstruction
  - aspiration of gastric contents
- Before interhospital transfer
  - neurological deterioration in transit
  - convulsions
  - unconscious patient (GCS <8)

Hypoventilation causes hypoxia and hypercarbia, and coughing and straining on an endotracheal tube increases intracranial pressure. Controlled hyperventilation to a P_aCO_2 of about 4 kPa is often used to control intracranial pressure, and neuromuscular blocking drugs are given, if required.

Hypotension results in reduced cerebral perfusion and adequate fluid replacement is essential. Closed head injury is never a cause of hypotension in adults and other factors must be sought.

Neurological assessment is undertaken with the Glasgow Coma Scale (GCS) (Box 29.3). Localising signs and pupillary reaction should additionally be sought and noted. Sequential changes in GCS score are a convenient way of assessing neurological progress. A GCS <8 is serious, and often an indication for endotracheal intubation.

Further management of the head-injured patient includes the use of intravenous mannitol (0·5 g/kg) which decreases intracranial pressure

Box 29.3   The Glasgow Coma Scale (GCS) Neurological assessment

Best Motor Response	
obeys commands	6
withdraws from painful stimuli	5
localises to painful stimuli	4
flexes to painful stimuli	3
extends to painful stimuli	2
no response	1
Best Verbal Response	
orientated	5
confused speech	4
inappropriate words	3
incomprehensible sounds	2
none	1
Eye Opening Response	
spontaneously	4
to speech	3
to pain	2
none	1

transiently. Anticonvulsants may be necessary if seizures occur, and antibiotics are used prophylactically in patients with compound skull fractures. Further advice can be obtained from the regional neurosurgical centre.

Patients are often transferred for neurosurgery. The decision whether to operate or not depends on the CT scans of the brain. Guidelines for transferring head-injured patients are shown in Box 29.4.

Box 29.4   Guidelines for transferring head-injured patients

- Physiological stabilisation before transfer
- Escorting doctor of adequate experience
- Appropriate drugs and equipment for transfer
- Intubated patients require:
  - sedation
  - paralysis
  - analgesia if indicated
- Use short acting drugs to allow neurological assessment
- Monitoring to minimal acceptable standard

161

Intubated patients should not increase intracranial pressure during transfer by coughing or straining, and hyperventilation is maintained. Short-acting drugs such as propofol, vecuronium, and fentanyl allow further assessment of the patient at the neurosurgical centre. A detailed handover to the receiving anaesthetist at the neurosurgical centre is essential.

Conclusion

The anaesthetist has a major role in the management of the head-injured patient, and the prevention of any secondary brain damage is the initial priority. Transfer of a patient with a head injury to a neurosurgical centre is not supposed to be undertaken by a novice trainee. However, this still occurs frequently, and if you have any doubts about the airway and/or neurological state, endotracheal intubation and ventilation is mandatory.

30: Anaesthesia in the corridor

Occasionally you will be asked to undertake anaesthesia away from the operating theatres. Inexperienced anaesthetists are not supposed to be involved with such work, as "playing away from home" is more hazardous. Within the hospital, anaesthetics may be given in:

- psychiatric unit for electroconvulsive therapy
- accident and emergency department
- coronary care unit
- radiology department.

Outside the hospital you may be asked to maintain anaesthesia during the transfer of patients between hospitals.

The principles and practice of safe anaesthesia remain the same regardless of the site. The essential requirements are shown in Box 30.1 and, if these are not met, the patient should be transferred to a safe environment. A senior anaesthetist must be called if any anaesthetic difficulty is anticipated. In general, anaesthesia needing a rapid sequence induction should be carried out in the main operating theatres.

Box 30.1   Minimum requirements for conduct of anaesthesia

- Qualified, experienced assistance
- Checked anaesthetic machine:
  - medical gas supplies
  - vaporisers
  - breathing systems
  - ventilator
- Adequate suction
- Adequate table tilt
- At least two working laryngoscopes
- Appropriate range of face masks, airways, endotracheal tubes
- Minimal monitoring equipment with alarms
- Appropriate drugs available
- Resuscitation drug box present
- Defibrillator working
- Appropriate recovery facilities and staff

Crises and complications can occur anywhere and you must be prepared. Do not be persuaded to work with inadequate facilities. Local medical staff can be very reassuring about the safety of anaesthesia over the last 20 years in some far corridor of the hospital.

Electroconvulsive therapy

Therapeutic convulsive therapy is used for the treatment of psychotic depression. The anaesthetist must consider the points shown in Box 30.2 in addition to the minimum requirements for the provision of anaesthesia.

Box 30.2   Considerations for electroconvulsive therapy anaesthesia

- Remote site anaesthesia
- Mental state of patient
- Modified convulsion
- Teeth protection
- Concomitant drug therapy
- Short duration procedure

After induction of anaesthesia, the convulsion is modified by the use of small doses of suxamethonium (25–50 mg) which make the patient apnoeic for a few minutes. Muscle pain after anaesthesia is not a major problem. The teeth must be protected by a mouth guard when the convulsion is applied. Since the anaesthetist must not touch the patient at the initiation of the convulsion, adequate oxygenation must be ensured before treatment.

Accident and emergency anaesthesia

The anaesthetist is a frequent visitor to the accident and emergency department to assist in cardiopulmonary resuscitation. Anaesthesia in this environment used to be common and was undertaken in difficult conditions; monitoring and recovery facilities were often non-existent. Both authors have been involved with "casualty lists"; these are hazardous for the patients and apparently character building for us.

Only if the basic requirements of safe anaesthesia are met (Box 30.1) should surgery occur. Anaesthesia is often challenging, for example for drainage of an abscess in an unpremedicated patient. If you have any doubt about the safety of the patient, surgery must be undertaken in the main operating theatres.

Radiological procedures

Again, the basic requirements of safe anaesthesia must be met. For scanning procedures, the anaesthetist often has to leave the patient and move to the scanning room, returning to monitor the patient physically between scans. You must be able to see the patient, either through a window, or by remote television, at all times. The monitoring equipment must always be clearly visible. In radiological procedures, the anaesthetic circuit is often 2–3 m long, and access to the airway and venous cannula is difficult during scanning.

Anaesthesia for cardioversion

Cardioversion is often undertaken in the coronary care unit where appropriate monitoring is usually available. This avoids the risks of moving a sick patient. Any subsequent arrhythmias are usually managed by the cardiologist. The minimum requirements for safe anaesthesia must be met. Often the procedure is of short duration and the cardioversion occurs under the induction dose of the intravenous agent.

Interhospital transfer of patients

The Association of Anaesthetists has produced guidelines on the monitoring requirements of patients undergoing anaesthesia, and these were discussed in Chapter 10. Similar requirements must be met when patients are transferred. Additional anaesthetic considerations are shown in Box 30.3.

Box 30.3   Anaesthetic considerations for patient transfer

- Medical condition of patient needing transfer
- Familiarity with equipment
- Secure airway and vascular access
- Drugs to manage transfer safely
- Appropriate monitoring
- Transfer to a suitable member of staff at receiving hospital

---

Patients should be physiologically stable before transfer. Ambulances often contain ventilators and suction equipment which are different from those found in hospitals. Familiarisation with these is essential before the patient is moved. Endotracheal tubes and intravenous cannulae must be secure. The correct drugs for the maintenance of anaesthesia, paralysis, and resuscitation must be available. A patient who is ventilated requires the same monitoring that is provided in theatre or the intensive care unit.

Conclusion

Beware of anaesthesia in some distant outpost of the hospital. If you have any doubts about the safety of the procedure, then insist that the patient is moved to the main operating theatres. Any inconvenience that this may cause is trivial when compared with the occurrence of an anaesthetic disaster.

Index

Page numbers in *italics* refer to tables and boxes and those in **bold** to figures that appear away from their text.